D1557473

PHYSICIAN-ASSISTED SUICIDE:
WHAT ARE THE ISSUES?

Philosophy and Medicine

VOLUME 67

Founding Co-Editor
Stuart F. Spicker

Editor

H. Tristram Engelhardt, Jr., *Department of Philosophy, Rice University, and Baylor College of Medicine, Houston, Texas*

Associate Editor

Kevin Wm. Wildes, S.J., *Department of Philosophy and Kennedy Institute of Ethics, Georgetown University, Washington, D.C.*

Editorial Board

The titles published in this series are listed at the end of this volume.

PHYSICIAN-ASSISTED SUICIDE: WHAT ARE THE ISSUES?

Edited by

LORETTA M. KOPELMAN
KENNETH A. DE VILLE

Department of Medical Humanities
The Brody School of Medicine at East Carolina University
Greenville, North Carolina
USA

KLUWER ACADEMIC PUBLISHERS
DORDRECHT / BOSTON / LONDON

Library of Congress Cataloging-in-Publication Data is available.

R
726
·P4975
2001

ISBN 0-7923-7142-9

Published by Kluwer Academic Publishers,
P.O. Box 17, 3300 AA Dordrecht, The Netherlands

Sold and distributed in North, Central and South America
by Kluwer Academic Publishers,
101 Philip Drive, Norwell, MA 02061, U.S.A.

In all other countries, sold and distributed
by Kluwer Academic Publishers, Distribution Center,
P.O. Box 322, 3300 AH Dordrecht, The Netherlands

Printed on acid-free paper

Printed and bound in Great Britain by MPG Books Ltd., Bodmin, Cornwall.

TABLE OF CONTENTS

PART IV: VISIONS OF THE FUTURE FOR
PHYSICIAN-ASSISTED SUICIDE

ACKNOWLEDGMENTS

It may seem surprising, even morbid, that the Department of Medical Humanities in the Brody School of Medicine at East Carolina University celebrated its twentieth anniversary with a conference on Physician-Assisted Suicide. Yet in many ways this topic represents the central goals of the department. It is an important topic that demands critical examination of moral, social and professional values and presuppositions about duty, relief of suffering, the limits of autonomy, compassion, nonmalificence, and fidelity. This subject, moreover, raises enduring problems about how to choose between such momentous values as preserving life and alleviating suffering when they conflict. Finally, this subject is timely since several important court cases were decided shortly before this conference was held on March 13-14, 1998 in Greenville, North Carolina, where most of the papers appearing herein were presented.

Only part of the conference was devoted to debates over physician-assisted suicide, the rest of the conference entitled, "Controversies in Bioethics," included papers on a variety of other topics. As the spring meeting of the Society of Health and Human Values (SHHV), it constituted very nearly its last event before it went out of existence. Later that year, SHHV along with two other organizations, the American Association of Bioethics and the Society for Bioethics Consultations, combined to form the American Society of Bioethics and Humanities (ASBH) in 1998. As the last president of the SHHV and the founding president of ASBH, the conference had special meaning for me (LMK). The conference was sponsored by the Department of Medical Humanities, the Bioethics Center, and the office of CME at the Brody School of Medicine.

It is our pleasure to acknowledge the contributions of several people who played key roles in the development of the Department of Medical Humanities and in enhancing the intellectual climate of the institution. We wish to thank the former Deans and Vice Chancellors for Health Sciences at the Brody School Medicine, William Laupus and James A. Hallock, for their support of the Department of Medicial Humanities. Dr. Laupus hired Loretta Kopelman in 1978 during the first year of the school's existence as a four-year medical school, enabling the program to grow with the school. He secured support for two more positions in the next six years and John Moskop and Todd Savitt joined the program. Reidar Lie was hired in 1987 and remained until he returned to Norway to head the medical humanities program at the University of Oslo. Jeff Kahn was appointed in 1989 and now directs the Center for Bioethics at the University of Minnesota. Kenneth De Ville was hired in 1992. In 1995, with the support of Dr. Hallock, the Pitt County Memorial Hospital funded the Bioethics Center in the Department of Medical Humanities at which time John Moskop became its director. Willem Landman was appointed that year, but returned to South Africa in 2000 as CEO of the Ethics Institute of South Africa. In 1998, David Resnik was hired. Our most recently hired faculty member in the Department is John Davis.

We wish to thank Lisa Boward Bagnell, administrator of the Department of Medical Humanities, for working so hard to collect the various draft essays from the authors and overseeing and attending to the many details of editing, proofreading, and formatting papers. Shirley Nett also helped with these tasks, as did our student assistant, Kristy L. Aro, a senior from East Carolina University's Department of English, who proofread the entire manuscript for us.

Most important, we would like to thank the contributors to this volume for their willingness to highlight the important issues that shape the debate over physician-assisted suicide.

Loretta M. Kopelman
Kenneth A. De Ville

July, 2001
Greenville, North Carolina

LORETTA M. KOPELMAN
KENNETH A. DE VILLE

THE CONTEMPORARY DEBATE OVER
PHYSICIAN-ASSISTED SUICIDE

The debate over physician-assisted suicide is momentous, complex, and contentious. Since ancient times reasonable and informed people of good will have disagreed about the permissibility of suicide, assisted suicide, and physician-assisted suicide and discussed the proper legal, ethical or professional response to people prepared to assist others with suicide or euthanasia. Some Hippocratic writings instructed early physicians about how to help patients who might wish to commit suicide or relieve their suffering through euthanasia. Yet the influential Hippocratic Oath from the same period forbids doctors from participating in such activities. Some philosophers, including Plato and Aristotle, offered principled objections to suicide or killing even for merciful reasons, while other early philosophers, most notably the Stoics, defended the rationality of such policies in some cases.

Contemporary societies are also strongly divided about the permissibility of suicide, assisted suicide, and physician-assisted suicide. Currently, few jurisdictions permit assisting suicides even where there are no criminal sanctions for attempting to commit suicide, and there is an almost universal prohibition against clinicians participating in euthanasia or assisting suicide. Yet recently The Netherlands and the state of Oregon began to allow physicians to assist suicides under some conditions, and The Netherlands and Japan have begun to permit euthanasia under certain circumstances. Some observers see this as a growing trend to develop more options for competent people who wish to end their lives.

After introducing recent court rulings that have had an impact on the contemporary U.S. debate over physician-assisted suicide, we consider the meaning of key terms in the discussion: assisted suicide, physician-assisted suicide, and euthanasia. In the final sections of this introduction, we offer a map of the main arguments for and against physician-assisted suicide and euthanasia.

Loretta M. Kopelman and Kenneth A. De Ville (eds.), Physician-Assisted Suicide, 1–25.
© 2001 *Kluwer Academic Publishers. Printed in Great Britain.*

1. TWO U.S. SUPREME COURT DECISIONS

Two rulings by the U.S. Supreme Court have altered the contemporary debate on physician-assisted suicide, *Washington v. Glucksberg* (1997) and *Vacco v. Quill* (1997). In these cases, decided together in June 1997, the Supreme Court unanimously reversed two circuit court decisions and upheld the constitutionality of state laws that prohibit assisted suicide, and therefore physician-assisted suicide. These much-anticipated rulings were, as many commentators realized, both an end and a beginning. In some ways, they mark the apex of over two decades of unprecedented litigation regarding end-of-life care. At the same time, however, *Glucksberg* and *Vacco* probably also signal the beginning of a new clinical, ethical, and legal debate over the extent of an individual's right to control the timing, manner and means of his or her death. After *Glucksberg* and *Vacco*, however, this debate will be more frequently relegated to state legislatures, rather than to the courts (Emanuel, 1998).

Although the issue of physician-aided death clearly has deep historic roots (Emanuel, 1994), the public and legal discussion of patients' rights in regard to end-of-life care exploded onto the scene primarily in the last two decades of the twentieth century. *In re Quinlan* (1976) and *Cruzan v. Director, Missouri Dept. of Health* (1990) captured the attention of the nation as well as the medical and bioethics communities. Since *Quinlan*, scores of state and federal appellate courts (and perhaps many more trial courts) have rendered judgments on the legal aspects of end-of-life decision making, most but not all relating to the appropriateness of the removal or refusal of life-sustaining medical treatment (National Center for State Courts, 1993). But public and professional discussion and interest did not remain limited to the removal or withholding of unwanted medical care. Increasingly, discussions of the defensibility of actively shortening lives no longer considered worth living crept into the public eye. For example, the activities of organizations such as the Hemlock society, as well as the popularity of its founder Derek Humphrey's book *Final Exit*, illustrate the way in which end-of-life discussions evolved and became central concerns of public debate and policy reform (Humphrey, 1991). Medical literature, too, gradually addressed with more regularity not only withdrawing care from patients who wished it, but also the more controversial questions of euthanasia and physician-assisted suicide, in articles such as the anonymous "It's Over Debbie," and Timothy Quill's narrative on death with dignity (Anonymous, 1988; Quill, 1991). Perhaps no one person played a greater role in publicizing and pressing the issue of physician-aided death than Jack Kevorkian, whose repeated and high profile forays into assisted suicide, as well as occasionally euthanasia, fed the increasingly restive public debate on the topics. By the early 1990s proposals favoring legally sanctioned physician aid-in-dying had been introduced in a number of states. In 1994, the electorate in Washington and California narrowly defeated proposals that would have legalized not only physician-assisted suicide, but also active euthanasia. In 1995, Oregon's Death with Dignity Law allowing physician-assisted suicide under circumscribed and regulated conditions became law (Or. Rev. Stat., 1995).

The *Glucksberg* and *Vacco* rulings should be viewed in the context of the two decades of activity that preceded them, but their implication and impact on the future of physician-aided death depends substantially on how they developed in the courts and how they were resolved.

A. Glucksberg

Glucksberg grew out of a challenge to a Washington felony statute that provided that: "A person is guilty of promoting suicide when he knowingly causes or aids another person to attempt suicide (Wash. Rev. Code 9A.36.060(1), 1994)."[1] In January 1994, Harold Glucksberg, and three other physicians who regularly treated suffering and terminally ill patients, challenged Washington's nearly 150-year criminal prohibition of assisted suicide. The physicians explained that they were prevented by threat of criminal prosecution from providing the treatment that would most benefit their patients. Glucksberg was also joined in the suit by three anonymous, terminal patients who wished their physicians' aid in dying, and by a non-profit organization which advocates physician-assisted suicide, Compassion in Dying. Glucksberg and the other plaintiffs claimed that there was a Fourteenth Amendment liberty interest "which extends to a personal choice by a mentally competent, terminally ill patient to commit physician-assisted suicide." They argued that a state's prohibition of assisted suicide placed "an undue burden" on that constitutionally protected liberty interest. The plaintiffs' legal argument relied heavily on *Cruzan* and *Planned Parenthood v. Casey* (Casey, 1992).

On May 3, 1994 federal district court judge Barbara Rothstein struck down the Washington law banning assisted suicide. She ruled that it violated the Due Process Clause of the Fourteenth Amendment because it placed an "undue burden" on a constitutionally protected liberty right (*Compassion in Dying*, 1994). Judge Rothstein declared that terminal, competent patients' liberty interests in access to assistance in ending their lives is constitutionally analogous to, and as compelling as, a pregnant woman's right to choose an abortion and an individual's right to refuse life-sustaining medical care. A three-judge panel of the Court of Appeals for the Ninth Circuit reversed Rothstein's ruling the next year (*Compassion in Dying*, 1995), but the full Circuit Court reheard the case *en banc* and affirmed the District Court's finding in favor of a right to assisted suicide (*Compassion in Dying*, 1996). In doing so, the Ninth Circuit declared that when considering terminally ill competent adults, "the Constitution encompasses a due process liberty interest in controlling the time and manner of one's death – that there is, in short, a constitutionally-recognized 'right to die' (*Compassion in Dying*, 1996 at 816)." According to the court, that constitutional liberty interest is unjustifiably limited by the state when physicians are not allowed to hasten patient deaths with medication.

The state of Washington appealed the ruling against its statute banning assisted suicide to the U.S. Supreme Court. By this point, public and professional interest had reached high levels. Over 60 *amicus curia* briefs were filed by public interest groups, bioethicists and philosophers on both sides of the assisted suicide debate, as well as by numerous state government agencies who wished to protect their own bans on assisted suicide. In *Glucksberg* the central legal question facing the Supreme Court was: Do mentally competent, terminally ill individuals have a fundamental liberty interest in access to the means of controlling the time and manner of their death that is protected by the Due Process Clause of the Fourteenth Amendment? The nature of the liberty interest defined by the court is important in this context. If the liberty interest is deemed "fundamental," then state action limiting that liberty is presumed unconstitutional and the state bears a heavy burden in justifying its limitation. However, if the liberty interest is not deemed "fundamental," then the state's action in limiting that liberty is presumed constitutional and upheld if the state regulation is merely rationally related to a legitimate government interest.[2] The case was argued before the Court on January 8, 1997. On June 26, 1997, the Supreme Court, in a 9-0 decision reversed the Ninth Circuit *Glucksberg* decision and ruled that state criminalization of assisted suicide was constitutionally permissible.

Justice William Rehnquist wrote the *Glucksberg* opinion which was joined by Justices O'Connor, Scalia, Kennedy, and Thomas. There were four concurring opinions.

The grounds upon which Fourteenth Amendment Due Process liberties are deemed "fundamental" are somewhat unsettled (Nowak and Rotunda, 1995, pp. 387-405), but the Court used a common two-part test. In order for a liberty to be fundamental and be granted the attendant protection, Rehnquist explained, it must be 1) "deeply rooted in this Nation's history and tradition," and 2) a "'careful description' of the asserted fundamental liberty interest (*Glucksberg*, 1997, p. 16)." Rehnquist defined the relevant asserted fundamental liberty as the "right to commit suicide which itself includes a right to assistance in doing so (*Glucksberg*, 1997, at p. 18)." Rehnquist then surveyed over 700 years of Anglo-American common law prohibition of assisted suicide including current criminal law. As a result, Rehnquist concluded that the asserted right has no place in the traditions of the country and to recognize such a right would reverse centuries of legal doctrine and practice as well as striking down the considered policy choice of virtually every state. Rehnquist rejected parallels drawn with the Court's findings in *Cruzan* and *Casey*. *Cruzan*, Rehnquist explained, was neither based on the right to control the manner and timing of one's death nor on a more general concept of personal autonomy. Instead, he contended that the right to refuse lifesaving hydration and nutrition is based on the well-established legal tradition that forced medication is battery and on that of protecting individual's decisions to refuse unwanted treatment. Similarly, Rehnquist dismissed parallels with *Casey* and the Court's other abortion precedents. Although the liberty interest recognized in *Casey* was personal, intimate, and important, according to Rehnquist, there was no suggestion in *Casey* that any and all such liberties would be elevated and given preferred constitutional protection. As a result, Rehnquist concluded that assistance in committing suicide is not a fundamental liberty interest protected by the Due Process Clause (*Glucksberg*, 1997, p. 23).

Having found that the asserted liberty right was not "fundamental," Rehnquist's remaining tasks were virtually perfunctory. A state regulation that limits a non-fundamental liberty interest need only be rationally related to a legitimate government interest. Under this standard of review courts must presume the constitutionality of the statute and must grant great deference to legislative judgments of fact. Those defending Washington's assisted suicide ban explained that it served a number of legitimate state interests. These interests include the same interests that courts typically weigh when balancing an individual's liberty interest in refusing unwanted life-sustaining medical treatment. In those cases, the state's interest is almost always found wanting. In contrast, the Court concluded that the state "unquestionably" had legitimate interests in prohibiting access to assisted suicide. Those state interests include: prohibiting intentionally killing and preserving human life; preventing suicide, especially among the vulnerable in the population; protecting the poor; protecting the integrity of the medical profession; and avoiding a possible slide toward voluntary or even involuntary euthanasia. Rehnquist was not required to weigh the relative strengths of each of these interests with precision since it was clear that they are legitimate and important, and that the law in question was at least reasonably related to their promotion and protection. As a result, the Court reversed the Ninth Circuit decision and concluded that Washington's ban on assisted suicide did not violate the Due Process Clause of the Fourteenth Amendment and could be enforced.

B. Vacco

At virtually the same time, but across the country, and on different constitutional grounds, *Vacco v. Quill* also worked its way toward the Supreme Court. In 1994, Timothy Quill, who had published a dramatic account of his dying patient, Diane, in the *New England Journal of Medicine*, two other physicians, and three terminally ill and suffering patients, challenged New York's assisted suicide statute. The New York statute stipulates that: "A person is guilty of manslaughter in the second degree when…he intentionally causes or aids another person to commit suicide (*N.Y. Penal Law* §125.15 (1987)." Unlike the litigants in Washington, Quill had actually faced legal action for his supposed role in the death of his patient, Diane. A state attorney general investigated Diane's death, but a New York grand jury refused to indict Quill. Quill and his fellow litigants' challenge claimed that although the prescription of lethal medication for mentally competent, terminally ill patients in great pain was consistent with the standards of their medical practice, they were deterred from providing such aid by the state's assisted suicide prohibition. Unlike in *Glucksberg*, the *Quill* litigants relied on the Equal Protection Clause of the Fourteenth Amendment. Simply stated, the Equal Protection Clause requires that state action must treat like cases alike but may treat unlike cases differently. If states do not, their action is subject to judicial scrutiny (*Plyler v. Doe*, 1982). The *Quill* litigants explained that it was well settled that individuals possessed a constitutional right to refuse medical treatment even if that refusal would result in their demise. Because such refusals were indistinguishable from physician-assisted suicide, they claimed, New York's assisted suicide ban violated the Equal Protection Clause. The trial judge at the District Court, however, disagreed, holding that "it is hardly unreasonable or irrational for the State to recognize a difference between allowing nature to take its course, even in the most severe situations, and intentionally using an artificial death-producing device." As a result, the District Court upheld New York's criminalization of assisted suicide (*Quill v. Koppell*, 1994).

The Court of Appeals for the Second Circuit reversed the District Court's finding and declared New York's ban on assisted suicide constitutionally void as a violation of the Equal Protection Clause of the Fourteenth Amendment. The court held that New York did *not* treat persons in a similar situation, i.e., all competent persons who are in the final stages of their illness, equally. The court reasoned that individuals with terminal illness who rely on life-support systems can end their lives and suffering by demanding the removal of this care. In contrast, individuals suffering from terminal and painful illnesses who do *not* rely on life-sustaining medical technology cannot end their lives and suffering by enlisting the aid of their physician in obtaining prescribed medication. The court found no significant difference between the ending of a life by the withdrawal of treatment, and the ending of a life by assisted suicide and so concluded that similarly situated groups of citizens were being treated dissimilarly by the law. The court then examined whether this dissimilar and unequal treatment by the state was rationally related to any legitimate state interest. The court concluded not, and overturned the statute (*Quill v. Koppell*, 1996).

The State of New York appealed the Circuit Court ruling in *Quill* to the U.S. Supreme Court. Oral arguments were held on the same day in January 1996 as those for *Glucksberg*. The Supreme Court handed down its ruling on the same day as *Glucksberg* and Chief Justice Rehnquist's majority opinion was joined by the same four justices offering concurrences. The Equal Protection Clause of the Fourteenth Amendment holds that no State shall "deny to any person within its jurisdiction the equal protection of the laws." As noted above, this prohibition has been interpreted to mean that states must treat like cases alike, but are allowed to treat unlike cases differently. Equal protection jurisprudence holds that as long as a particular state action or legislation does not adversely affect a fundamental right or target a suspect class (a classification based on race, ethnicity or alienage) or "quasi suspect" class (gender or age), it will be upheld as long as it is rationally related to a legitimate state goal (Nowak and Rotunda, 1995, pp. 597–611).[3] Rehnquist's majority opinion in *Quill* reviewed these standards and noted that New York's assisted suicide statute did not infringe on a fundamental right (a notion reinforced by the *Glucksberg* decision handed down the same day) nor did it involve a so-called "suspect" classification. As a result, the Court was required to give a strong presumption of validity to the state action and it need only pass the rational-relation test.

Moreover, Rehnquist contended that, on the face of it, New York's ban on assisted suicide discriminated against no single group. "*Everyone*, regardless of physical condition, is entitled, if competent, to refuse unwanted lifesaving medical treatment, *no one* is permitted to assist a suicide (*Quill* 1997, p. 4*)*." Rehnquist then responded to the Circuit Court's contention that refusing life-sustaining medical treatment "is nothing more or less than assisted suicide." The majority opinion reasoned that the distinction is widely recognized in both medical and legal traditions and thus supported a sufficiently rational distinction upon which a state legislature can distinguish one action from another. In fact, Rehnquist noted that the New York legislature specifically stated in its Do Not Resuscitate Order statute that such practices, though allowable, are "not intended to promote suicide, assisted suicide, or euthanasia (N.Y. Public Health Law, 1994)." Rehnquist concluded that these considerations, legal and medical traditions and contemporary practice support constitutional and judicial deference to New York's judgment that the two acts are different. The legislature's reasons for treating the two actions differently echoed the state concerns that were discussed and endorsed in *Glucksberg*: protecting human life; preventing suicide; maintaining physicians' role as healers; protecting vulnerable individuals, etc. Giving deference to this legislative determination, Rehnquist concluded that these "valid and important public interests easily satisfy the constitutional requirement that a legislative classification bear a rational relation to some legitimate end (*Quill* 1997, p. 12)."

Along with *Glucksberg* and *Quill*, the 1997 Supreme Court refused to review *Lee v. Oregon*, the Ninth Circuit ruling which held that Oregon's Death with Dignity act did not violate the Equal Protection Clause of the

Fourteenth Amendment. Together, these cases suggest that physician assisted suicides are neither constitutionally prohibited nor constitutionally required and that the most important constitutional issues regarding physician-assisted suicide have now been resolved.

C. Critics of Glucksberg and Quill

A number of court observers and advocates of physician-assisted suicide, however, have attacked the majority's reasoning in *Glucksberg* and *Quill* and pointed to numerous comments in the concurring opinions which they believe suggest that the constitutional battle over assisted suicide may not yet be over. Several commentators have argued, for example, that Rehnquist's designation of the relevant liberty interest as one of the "right to suicide" rather than the "right to control the manner and time" of one's death significantly affected the results of the Court's subsequent constitutional analysis and final decision (Tucker, 1998, p. 926). It is reasonable to suggest that Rehnquist's narrow articulation of the relevant right under consideration made it more difficult to find evidence for its support in the jurisprudence and traditions of the country sufficient for the Court to deem it "fundamental." There is, after all, little support culturally or legally in Anglo-American culture and law for legalized and aided suicide. In contrast, there has been an escalating and dramatic increase culturally and legally in the recognition of individual autonomy, especially in issues that relate to bodily integrity, life, death and conception. Such evidence would have lent credence to the *Glucksberg* and *Quill* contention that society and the court should recognize a fundamental right in controlling the manner and timing of one's death.

The argument that individuals should have a general, constitutionally protected interest in making judgments about their death was vigorously and eloquently outlined by the so-called "philosophers' brief" submitted by a "dream team" of contemporary philosophers (Dworkin et al., 1997). Significantly, the Court neither mentioned the "philosophers' brief" nor directly engaged its arguments in debate. Given that the majority decision addressed the far narrower question of a right to assistance in suicide, the omission is not surprising. Such arguments, however, would be of far more relevance if the issue under consideration was the broader one of generalized individual autonomy. Whether the mere rephrasing of the relevant right to be considered would have been sufficient to capture the votes of five justices and reverse the outcome of two unanimous decisions is uncertain. It is perhaps equally likely, in fact, that the Court would have been *more* hesitant to approve a broader fundamental right, instead of one that was limited merely to assistance in suicide for terminally ill patients.

Other critics of Rehnquist's majority opinion in *Glucksberg* and *Quill* and supporters of legalized assisted suicide suggest that while the 9–0 decision slammed a door on assisted suicide, the concurring opinions left open a window. Some commentators, for example, find evidence in the concurring opinions of Justice O'Connor and others that if a future case were based on other, more narrow, grounds, then the Court might be willing to entertain the existence of a right to physician-assisted suicide. Specifically, several concurring opinions suggested that there may be a constitutionally protected right to die free from avoidable pain. If such a right existed, state law could not bar an individual access to the means of controlling or ending his or her pain. Accordingly, if ending one's life was the only means of ending one's pain, then assisted suicide might be a protected activity under those conditions (e.g., Burt, 1997; Gostin, 1997).

Those making this argument may face several legal and conceptual obstacles. Such language in the concurrances is just as likely to mean that individuals may have a constitutional remedy if the state denies them access to adequate pain control, either through an inappropriate prosecution of a so-called double-effect case or through excessively onerous narcotic control regulation. Even if the concurrence language relating to a right to control one's pain does encompass a potential right to assisted suicide, that right will likely be extraordinarily narrow and rarely invoked. Consider the conditions under which such a constitutional case would arise. A physician would have to provide aid in dying to a patient, face criminal charges and be convinced of manslaughter or murder. His or her constitutional defense would be based on the claim that individuals possess a constitutionally protected right to die free of pain even if that entails suicide or assisted suicide. If a court accepted the physician's constitutional claim the conviction would be overturned. Other physicians would then know that such a defense *might* work in court. The key issue, however, is that such a constitutional challenge would almost always be an "as applied" challenge (as opposed to a "facial" challenge of the statue itself) which is limited only to the imposition of the statute prohibiting assisted suicide in this particular case or type of case. It is unlikely that such a precedent would provide blanket protection *prospectively* to a broad range of physicians who wished to end their patients' lives to end their pain. Subsequent physicians would also likely have to act to aid their patients at the bedside, and face prosecution, without the guarantee of constitutional protection under the particular factual scenario at hand. Thus, while there is textual evidence in the concurrances that might inform future constitutional challenges regarding the individual prosecution of physicians for physician-assisted suicide, it seems unlikely to result in a broad-based acknowledgement of a constitutional right to physician-assisted suicide that will affect a large number of physicians and patients.

D. The Laboratories of the States

Some top constitutional scholars still see a significant constitutional future for physician-assisted suicide based upon credible readings of the various concurring opinions (Levinson, 1997). Despite their intellectual plausibility, however, they remain speculative and should not distract from the relatively unambiguous short-term impact of *Glucksberg* and *Quill*, which is to refer the decision regarding physician-assisted suicide to the so-called laboratory of the states (Kamisar, 1998). The advisability and wisdom of relegating the assisted-suicide debate to the legislative branch of government will ultimately depend on whether the courts or legislatures are better equipped to deal with the relevant issues more effectively. Legislatures are often effective fact-finding and debating forums in which to develop policy that will most benefit society and best reflect the public will.

Those who favor physician-assisted suicide should not despair. Many of the arguments that failed at the constitutional level may find more success in the court of public opinion. Constitutional jurisprudence is not always sensitive to or compatible with the distinctions, insights and arguments offered by moral philosophy. For example, the relatively common philosophical discussions regarding the moral distinction between acts and omissions, as well as the grand defense of individual autonomy presented in the "philosophers' brief," were ignored in the constitutional discussion by the *Glucksberg* and *Quill* court. Such philosophical guidance, however, may be relevant and useful in the policy-related debates that should take place in determining whether a state should allow or prohibit physician-assisted suicide. Nor, obviously, should opponents of the practice fear legislative control over physician-assisted suicide. A legislatively created "right" to assistance in dying would almost certainly be easier to limit and monitor than a constitutionally mandated right to control the timing, manner and details of one's death.

Legislative action is clearly not inerrant. Legislation action results not only from reasoned deliberation but also from compromise and political pressure as well. Because interest group activity often plays a significant role in legislative motivation, resulting legislation does not always take the interests and rights of all affected parties fully into consideration. In addition, the unintended consequences of legislation are legion, especially in the health care setting where technology, demographics, and delivery mechanisms change almost monthly. The twin faults of vagueness on one hand, and hyper-specificity on the other, are endemic to statutory law – especially that related to medical care, which by its nature remains a case-by-case endeavor. But, these observations should not be read as a condemnation of the legislative mandate to explore and regulate aid in dying. Instead, they should underscore the difficulty of the endeavor and signal the need for careful, sensitive and full consideration of the theoretical, conceptual, philosophical as well as the practical implications of all policy options regarding physician-assisted suicide.

2. KEY CONCEPTS IN AN ANCIENT DEBATE

The debate over physician-assisted suicide is, in part, conceptual, or about how to understand what is entailed by such notions as "right to control one's destiny" and "the duty to comfort people." In this section we focus upon the sometimes-contentious debate over the meaning of some key locutions in this discussion: suicide, assisted suicide, physician-assisted suicide, and euthanasia.

A *suicide* will be understood as the voluntary and intentional taking of one's own life. People who cannot tolerate their lives may commit suicide by taking poisons, slitting their wrists, crashing their cars, or leaping from bridges. But according to this definition, police, firemen and soldiers who heroically sacrifice themselves also commit suicide, albeit for very different reasons. They do not wish to die, but to save others. Some reject this definition of "suicide" simply because they believe that acts of suicides should be limited to ignoble deeds. The philosopher Immanuel Kant, for example, denies the solder's act of sacrifice is a suicide because it is virtuous. Making acts of suicide wrong by definition, however, entirely discounts the arguments that have persuaded many people since ancient times that suicide and assisted suicide can sometime be justifiable. Thus we offer this more neutral definition. Those with principled objections to physician-assisted suicide often believe suicide is self-murder and evil in itself. This view is less common today, although one cannot assume that if suicide is permissible then assisting in a suicide should also be permitted (Holmes, 2000).

An *assisted suicide* occurs when someone, by act or omission, helps another person end his or her life voluntarily and intentionally. In the clear cases, all parties unambiguously convey their intentions and each person involved makes a voluntary, competent and informed choice. The individual who assists in a suicide does not kill the person directly but helps the person kill himself/herself. Assistance can take various forms including providing the means, such as arsenic, removing some obstacle, such as a restraint, or refraining from doing something, such as locking a cabinet. *Physician-assisted suicide* occurs when a physician gives assistance to enable someone to bring about his/her own death. To count as a suicide, the person must be the agent of his/her own death, unlike euthanasia.

Euthanasia, sometimes called *mercy killing*, occurs when someone terminates the life of another person for compassionate reasons. "Euthanasia" comes from the Greek and means a good death, or *eu* (good) and thanatos (death). Defenders of euthanasia distinguish *active euthanasia* (killing someone deliberately and for compassionate reasons) from *passive euthanasia* (allowing someone to die). Critics argue that the acts of killing and letting die are sufficiently different that it is misleading to use the same word to describe both, and generally contrast active euthanasia with the locution-letting die. Critics and defenders agree that passive euthanasia/letting die is sometimes morally justifiable, but disagree about whether a policy permitting active euthanasia is ever prudent to adopt.

Considerable attention has been paid to the question of whether active euthanasia and passive euthanasia/letting die are really different, either conceptually or morally. Some attempts to distinguish them are framed in terms of: 1) acts vs. omissions, 2) ordinary treatment vs. extraordinary treatment, 3) withdrawing treatment vs. withholding treatment, 4) whether the cause of death is the intervention or some underlying pathology, and 5) whether the patient requests some intervention or refuses a life-sustaining treatment.[4] These same issues can also be important in the physician-assisted suicide debate. As noted, some of these distinctions are used by the U.S. Supreme Court rules in ruling in *Glucksberg* and *Vacco* in trying to distinguish standard medical care from physician-assisted suicide.

Most commentators agree that these distinctions fail to differentiate sharply active from passive means whether it is in reference to differentiating active euthanasia from passive euthanasia/letting die or physician-assisted suicide from standard medical care. They disagree, however, about what conclusion to draw from this. Some people argue the fuzzy borders between these concepts show that, where passive euthanasia/letting die is permissible, then so is active euthanasia, and that where standard of care allows a double effect to be permissible then so is physician-assisted suicide. There are disputes about what sort of pain relief is standard, especially where giving a patient adequate pain relief may hasten his or her death. There are also disagreements about what medication, hydration or nutrition may be withheld or withdrawn, and whether this is fundamentally different from physician-assisted suicide (Frey, 2000). Others claim that the lack of a sharp distinction justifies forbidding them all. Still others argue that the lack of a bright line between them does not show that distinctions are not useful for many purposes any more that the lack of a sharp boundary between night and day makes those concepts useless (Kopelman, 2000).

Further distinctions are made based upon whether the euthanasia is voluntary, nonvoluntary or involuntary. Voluntary active euthanasia occurs when the person consents, perhaps even requests, the mercy killing. If euthanasia is performed but the person never consented because he or she is a child, incompetent, or was never consulted, it is a case of *nonvoluntary active euthanasia. Involuntary active euthanasia* is a questionable category since it would occur if the person objects to being killed but the act were really for the person's good. Some commentators find it hard to imagine involuntary "euthanasia" being an act of mercy and not simply murder, especially in medical settings. This category presupposes not only that the killer knows that the person is about to suffer a horrible fate but that killing the person over his or her objections would be justifiable and merciful in the face of the person's protests. Suppose that a pilot crashes his plane and begs for help because he wants to live. No equipment is available to help him, and fire is rapidly engulfing the aircraft. Some people would argue that killing the pilot would be an act of mercy. Other commentators would argue that higher duties override mercy in such cases.

The definitions of the key terms and concepts, then, are not wholly independent of the debates over the permissibility of suicide, assisted suicide, physician-assisted suicide, or euthanasia. Those with different views about their permissibility tend to provide somewhat different analyses. We have rejected those definitions that make these activities either right or wrong by definition.

3. KEY ARGUMENTS FOR PHYSICIAN-ASSISTED SUICIDE

The debate over physician-assisted suicide is intertwined with questions about the permissibility of suicide, assisted suicide, voluntary active euthanasia/mercy killing, and passive euthanasia/letting die. Part of the discussion about physician-assisted suicide concerns the degree to which these four categories call for distinct moral, clinical, social or legal responses. The responses can be divided into those who defend physician-assisted suicide and those who object. But those who object may do so on either of two grounds: *principled* grounds, i.e., they regard these activities as wrong in all circumstances or on *nonprincipled* grounds, i.e., they do not believe these activities are always wrong but that, given the circumstances, more prudent, less disruptive or more effective policies exist.

A. Liberty arguments

For some commentators the most powerful and persuasive argument for legalizing physician-assisted suicide concerns increasing people's liberty (Dworkin et al., 1997; Brock, 2001; Battin, 2001). On this view, the proper response to our ancient disagreements about how to face suffering, pain and death is to permit people to choose the sort of assistance in dying that best suits them. Competent, rational, and informed individuals may decide that their lives are no longer worth living and want to plan the time and circumstance of their death. In their view, maximizing options for people defends their distinct perspectives and interests, protecting them from social manipulation. These are negative rights, or rights not to be interfered with, and do not affect others.[5] None are required to participate if they do not wish.

Defenders of legalizing physician-assisted suicide favor allowing these actions by willing parties. They do not wish, for example, to require the unwilling doctor to assist a patient who requests help committing suicide. Even in cultures where euthanasia and assisted suicide were openly practiced, a justification had to be given for such proceedings. As we saw, Epictetus argued that people had to show first that such acts were rational.

People should decide how to end their own lives when it is intolerable to them, on this view; their actions typically affect no one else, and usually this option allows the person to avoid suffering or what is to them a humiliating or dishonorable existence. Allowing people to have a free choice about the sort of assistance in dying they choose acknowledges that this is a personal matter and shows respect for people's autonomy or rights of self-determination. Consequently, the argument continues, we should respect people's choices and allow them to exercise their autonomy by permitting important options. Policy and research should try to enhance people's choices regarding assistance in dying and include not only good advance care planning, palliative care and withdrawal of life-sustaining treatments, but, they conclude, also assisted suicide or physician-assisted suicides.

With sufficient safeguards, physician-assisted suicide not only honors people's rights of self-determination but, defenders hold, can be prudent policy. They favor an array of safeguards to ensure that people make an informed, unforced, and rational decision, typically including that the person is terminally ill and competent, and that other physicians confirm the diagnosis, prognosis and approve the request. Those defending physician-assisted suicide generally argue that doctors are needed as counselors to assure that the choice is not only informed but also unforced, and competent or rational.

Some carry the liberty argument farther, arguing that even these restrictions are unjustifiable infringements on people's freedom. For example, they question why people must be terminally ill to obtain relief, pointing out that the claims of people with degenerative diseases may sometimes be at least as compelling. Anecdotal evidence indicates that people may seek active euthanasia/mercy killing, assisted suicide, or physician-assisted suicide not only to avoid the last stages of terminal illnesses, but also to avoid mental and physical deterioration from long term, chronic and progressive diseases such as Alzheimer's and Huntington's diseases (Povar, 2001). These are most anguishing to patients in the initial stages when they are relatively functional and most disturbing to the family when patients are ravaged by these diseases. People in the early stages sometimes request assistance in dying from clinicians when they reach a certain stage of anticipated deterioration. While they do not want to die while they have some facilities, they fear waiting too long until they lack capacity to kill themselves.

Some do not think this policy goes far enough. They question why the individual should have to be competent to have this right; if competent people have a right not to suffer, why should incompetent people not have this right as well? (Landman, 2001). Other persons normally can assert liberty-rights on behalf of incompetent persons, and these commentators favor acknowledging that both competent and incompetent people have this right. Still other commentators question why physicians alone should have this authority to assist in suicide and regard it to be an unwarranted restriction of people's liberty.

B. Relief of Suffering as a Basis for Physician-Assisted Suicide

Another argument used to support the permissibility of physician-assisted suicide concerns the duty to relieve suffering or the importance of treating others with compassion. An important goal of medicine is to relieve suffering, and in some cases it overrides the goal of prolonging life. One reason to give authority to doctors for assisted suicide, defenders argue, emanates from physicians' long-standing duties to relieve suffering. Many of the best-known accounts of physician-assisted suicide are cases where compassionate, knowledgeable, and understanding physicians believed their duty to assist in a suicide in order to relieve pain, anguish or suffering was a higher duty than prolonging life (Quill, 1991; Anonymous, 1988).

C. No Moral Difference Between Physician-Assisted Suicide and Permissible Activities

Some commentators argue that it is unreasonable to permit passive euthanasia/withholding treatment while prohibiting physician-assisted suicide because there is no genuine moral difference between them. Society and the courts now agree that competent people have a right to forgo life-saving treatment and get adequate pain medication even if that hastens their death. This "no moral difference argument" takes two forms. First, some commentators argue that we cannot draw a bright line between those acts that have social approval and assisted suicide or euthanasia and there are practical difficulties about distinguishing them.

If we cannot draw a bright line between those acts that have social approval and assisted suicide, then if the one is a morally permissible social policy, the other ought to be as well. This reasoning is problematic. It is an argument from gradualism holding that in the absence of clear lines to separate two or more things, they are fundamentally the same thing. The difficulty with this kind of argument from gradualism is that we can sometimes use paradigms and other markers to make meaningful distinctions. There is no clear mark between the notes of C and D or between orange and red yet they can be differentiated.

There is a second and more plausible version of the "no-moral-difference" argument. Some commentators argue that there is no moral difference between doctors' acts and omissions in assisting someone to hasten death since both are actions that may be justifiable or not, depending upon the circumstances. The key moral difference between those that are and are not justifiable is unrelated to using active or passive means (Rachels, 1975). Unless one defends a principled objection to assisted suicide, it is generally acknowledged that there are cases where assisted suicide would be justifiable.

4. PRINCIPLED ARGUMENTS AGAINST PHYSICIAN-ASSISTED SUICIDE

Some object to physician-assisted suicide, as well as assisted suicide and active euthanasia, because they hold that these activities are always wrong, no matter what the circumstances. These are principled objections and they take several different forms. Some commentators argue that the person who commits suicide or assists another, destroys what properly belongs to God or the gods. Plato, Aquinas, and Kant took the view that our lives are not ours to dispose of since we belong to God. Immanuel Kant writes, "We have been placed in this world under certain conditions and for specific purposes. Thus, suicide opposes the purpose of his creator; he arrives in the other world as one who has deserted his post; he must be looked upon as a rebel against God" (Kant, 1930 [1774], p. 154). Locke, in the *Second Treatise on Civil Government* also argued that people are the property of God and cannot quit their station without permission (Locke, 1690, paragraph 6). Aristotle argued that suicide was a crime against the state in depriving the polis of a citizen.

Still another principled argument is that a suicide, and thus assisting a suicide, degrades humanity by treating people as disposable things rather than persons. Kant also defended this argument, maintaining that doing one's duty is the highest good. Soldiers who die in battle for the sake of comrades are not suicides at all, but, according to Kant, performing their duty and simply a victim of fate. Clearly Kant wanted to distinguish between the sacrifices we consider noble from those which he regarded as an evasion of duty.

Yet another principled argument concerns the act of suicide being opposed to nature. A suicide, according to this argument, should be viewed as unnatural. Aquinas argued that self-destruction is contrary to the natural and genuine feelings of human beings to love and preserve themselves. It is horrendous, unnatural and an extreme form of self-mutilation.

Principled objections were widely attacked by enlightenment philosophers such as David Hume. These critics leveled such devastating assaults on each of these principled arguments that their over-all influence has lessened (Edwards, 1998). Critics questioned assumptions that a merciful God would want creatures to suffer torments for no purpose. They also argued that it is degrading to live in certain circumstances. The notion of what is or is not "natural" is controversial and often shaped to the desired conclusion. These and other arguments against principled objections shifted the discussion. Considerably more attention is now paid to nonprincipled objections that such activities are imprudent or that other more effective and less disruptive means exist, rather than principled objections.

5. NONPRINCIPLED OR CONTINGENT OBJECTIONS TO PHYSICIAN-ASSISTED SUICIDE

Commentators who defend *nonprincipled objections* to permitting physician-assisted suicide do not regard this assistance as always and invariably wrong. They do not regard such activities to be invariably bad because they are always sinful, immoral, unnatural, sick, or against God's will. Rather, defenders of nonprincipled objections agree that these activities might sometimes be justifiable, but argue more effective and less disruptive, contentious or dangerous policy options can achieve the desired ends. They concede, however, that circumstances might change.

Nonprincipled objections take several different forms. Some commentators may argue that the social costs are too high, because, for example, physician-assisted suicide would be likely to undermine quests for better pain management, social support, solidarity or important clinical values (Singer and Seigler, 1990; Zoloth, 2001). Some suggest that physician-assisted suicide raises troubling issues in a medical climate where for-profit managed care organizations seem to challenge traditional clinical values. Defenders, however, deny that these are the likely consequences of a good physician-assisted suicide policy (Brock, 2001; Battin, 2001; Landman, 2001; Deville, 2001). In what follows we discuss three nonprincipled objections to physician-assisted suicide based upon there being more effective and less disruptive means to achieve the same ends, or that the social costs for physician-assisted suicide are too high.

A. Liberties to Refuse Medical Interventions, Food and Water

People have the liberty to refuse medical interventions, as we have seen. In some but not all jurisdictions they can also refuse hydration and nutrition. Gert, Culver, and Clouser (1998) argue that permitting people to refuse medication would be a good general policy and undercut the need for physician-assisted suicide. They argue that we must carefully distinguish between valid refusals and valid requests, and should honor their valid refusals of medications, food and water. This would be a less disruptive and more effective policy than permitting physician-assisted suicide. Among the chief obstacles to its adoption, commentators argue, are misconceptions that dying by dehydration or starvation is cruel or painful. An advantage is that such a policy would almost certainly be more efficient than policies with their build-in safeguards permitting physician-assisted suicide or active euthanasia. This is because in all likelihood death from dehydration would occur within two weeks, but it might be longer to negotiate and fulfill the various legal and institutional safe-guards and reviews favored by advocates of assisted suicide or physician-assisted suicide. Adopting such a policy has several advantages. It need not be restricted to terminal patients, as is often the case with policies written favoring physician-assisted suicide. It further enhances people's options by its very gradualism in allowing people to reflect and reconsider their choice as the process is set in motion (Kopelman, 2001).

B. Better Palliative, Pain and Other Care

Many, perhaps most, people seeking assisted suicide, physician-assisted suicide or active voluntary euthanasia would want to live if their situation were improved. Defenders argue that we should not consider physician-assisted suicide or active euthanasia while many options exist to improve the situation of those in need of help (Resnik, 2001; Kopelman, 2001). This includes better social support, pain management and palliative care. Good palliative care provides a compassionate response and therefore neutralizes at least one powerful argument for assisted suicide, physician-assisted suicide or active voluntary euthanasia concerning duties to relieve suffering or the importance of treating others with compassion. Arguably some would still request assistance in dying by means of assisted suicide or active euthanasia, even if they were not in pain, but studies show most would not want to die if the quality of their lives improved.

C. Critics of Liberty Arguments and Liberalism

Some commentators attack the liberty argument for legalizing assisted suicide (and for physician-assisted suicide, or voluntary active euthanasia). These critics argue that such policies are too extreme in focusing so exclusively upon liberty rights and individualism (Zoloth, 2001). On this view, such policies mistakenly detach people from the web of their social commitments, considering them as separate social units entirely free to make self-regarding behavior. Failing to appreciate the social context of people's lives promotes the view that people ought to be able to get what they want, despite social costs. Rather people should be seen as part of a network of relationships and necessarily members of communities. Personal interest alone might dictate that someone has an interest in wishing for assistance in suicide (or active euthanasia), but this does not settle whether their preferences should be honored or if it is a prudent social policy to offer these options.[6]

For example, given the number of people who are uninsured or denied basic care, resources would be better used for other purposes. But defenders of physician-assisted suicide argue it would not be more costly and might even be cost effective for a society. This response raises another concern that these actions might be encouraged to save money rather than to answer people's need for assistance in dying. Some minority groups fear such a stance. And whether or not they are right, studies show that alarming biases exist in the way life-saving and costly therapies are allocated to patients. For reasons of community solidarity, they conclude, we should not permit physician-assisted suicide (or assisted suicide or voluntary active euthanasia). Many groups have strong views about these means and others are fearful of the health care systems. For them such options may undermine social solidarity. Some commentators charge that the appeal to autonomy rights in the physician-assisted suicide debate is spurious because it has separated from the moral and social basis for liberty rights (Zoloth, 2001).

Defenders reject the characterization of the liberalism given by these critics of policies legalizing assisted suicide (or physician-assisted suicide, or voluntary active euthanasia) as excessively individualistic (Battin, 2001; Brock, 2001). With proper protections, they hold, it is just and beneficial to promote the form of assistance in dying that people wish; since these liberties do not harm others, are not excessively individualistic, do not promote unreasonable self-interested requests given social resources, and do not undermine compassionate responses to people. Defenders argue that education may be the key to patients' and others' understanding that withholding and withdrawing of lifesaving treatment is fundamentally similar to the proposals they defend. Extending options in dying, they argue, further enhances a patient's autonomy and best interest; it is not to save money. The new laws in Oregon and policies in the Netherlands may help us assess these practical concerns about how to evaluate these nonprincipled concerns about physician-assisted suicide (or assisted suicide or voluntary active euthanasia). Some commentators, however, question if these new laws will deeply affect medical practice (DeVille, 2001).

Critics and defenders of liberalism continue to debate whether liberal conceptions of personal autonomy (1) are necessarily too individualistic, (2) undermine compassionate responses to people, especially those whose requests might be imprudent, ill informed, incompetent, or nonautonomous, or (3) promotes unreasonable self-interested requests given social resources.

6. CONCLUSION

We have tried to introduce the assumptions, principles and concerns about physician-assisted suicide. If suicide is permissible, why should people be prohibited from assisting in a suicide? And if assisting suicide is permissible, why should physicians alone be authorized to assist people? Moreover, if withholding or withdrawing life-saving treatments is approved under some circumstances, why should active euthanasia be forbidden? Answering these questions raises fundamental issues about the value of life, the worth of a person to his/her community, rights of self-determination, duties of clinicians to relieve suffering, and the meaning of life itself. Finally, some commentators are skeptical that these disputes can ever be solved rationally because the debate is so intertwined with choices about the nature of our rights, duties and of morality itself (Engelhardt, 2001). Whether this creates unbridgeable chasms among us remains to be seen.

Brody School of Medicine at East Carolina University
Greenville, North Carolina

NOTES

[1] Washington state law specifically stipulated that the "withholding or withdrawal of life-sustaining treatment" at the request of a competent patient was not a criminal act (Wash. Rev. Code, Sec. 70. 122.070 (1).

[2] State actions reviewed under the former standard are rarely upheld, and those under the latter standard are very rarely overturned.

[3] Legislation that burdens a fundamental right is presumed unconstitutional by the Court and permitted only if it is necessary to fulfill a compelling state interest and that the means the legislature used are narrowly tailored to meet that end. This "strict scrutiny" test is extraordinarily difficult to meet.

[4] Briefly, consider some of the problems with them. First, what is ordinary or extraordinary is very much tied to contingencies such as resources and the patient's condition, so it offers little aid in determining what is in general a compassionate or dutiful response. Second, deliberate omissions, such as not turning on a respirator, are also actions and, once again fail to address the pertinent questions of the justifiability or compassion of the act. Third, beginning a treatment and then withdrawing it may feel different from failing to begin a treatment, but the issue is whether giving it is needed, compassionate or a duty; the issue is not if or when it is initiated. Similarly, the fourth attempt to distinguish them fails to address whether providing something is a duty or compassionate response; a treatable chronic illness may be life-threatening without treatment, so this distinction may focus upon what seems

irrelevant. Finally, some patients are unable to request euthanasia because they are not or never were competent so the fifth attempt also fails.

[5] Ikonomidis and Singer, for example, claim liberalism should be understood as, "expressed in terms of negative freedom, rank-order desires, personal identification, and, notably, historical formulation which highlights the broad social embeddedness of the individual." (Ikonomidis and Singer, 1999, p. 523).

[6] For example, many feminists and communitarians have rejected what they view as the atomistic conception of moral agency inherent in liberalism.

REFERENCES

Anonymous: 1988, 'A piece of my mind. It's over, Debbie', *The Journal of the American Medical Association* 259, 272.

Aristotle: 4th Century, *Nicomachaen Ethics* 1138a, 6–14.

Battin, M.P.: 2001, 'Safe, legal, rare? Physician-assisted suicide and cultural change in the future', this volume, 187–201.

Battin, M.P.: 1982, *Ethical Issues in Suicide*, Engelwood Cliffs, NJ: Prentice Hall.

Brock, D.W.: 2001, 'Physician-assisted suicide-the worry about abuse', this volume, 59–74.

Burt, R.: 1997, 'The Supreme Court speaks: not assisted suicide but a right to palliative care', *The New England Journal of Medicine* 337, 1234–1236.

Compassion in Dying v. Washington, 850 F. Supp. 1454 (W.D. Wash. 1994).

Compassion in Dying v. Washington, 49 F.3d 586 (9th Cir. 1995).

Compassion in Dying v. Washington, 79 F.3d 790 (9th Cir. 1996).

Cruzan v. Director, Missouri Dept. of Health, 497 U.S. 261, 110 S. Ct. 2841 (1990).

Humphreys, D.: 1997, *Final Exit: The Practicalities of Self-Deliverance and Assisted Suicide for the Dying.* Denver, Colorado: The Hemlock Society.

De Ville, K.A.: 2001, 'Physician-assisted suicide and the states: short-, medium-, and long-term', this volume, 171–186.

Dworkin, R. *et al.*: 1997, 'Assisted suicide: the philosophers' brief', *New York Review of Books* 44, 41–47.

Edwards, P.: 1998, 'The ethics of suicide', *Rutledge Encyclopedia of Philosophy,* New York.

Elliot, C.: 1996, 'Philosopher assisted suicide and euthanasia', *British Medical Journal* 313, 1088–1089.

Emanuel, E.J.: 1994, 'The history of euthanasia debates in the United States and Britain', *Annals of Internal Medicine* 121, 793–802.

Emanuel, E.J.: 1998, 'The future of euthanasia and physician-assisted suicide: beyond rights talk to informed public policy', *Minnesota Law Review* 82: 983–1014.

Engelhardt, H.T., Jr.: 2001, 'Physician-assisted suicide and euthanasia: another battle in the culture wars', this volume, 29–41.

Frey, R.G.: 2001, 'Refusals/withdrawals and physician-assisted suicide', this volume, 43–57.

Gert, B. et al.: 1998, 'An alternative to physician-assisted suicide: a conceptual and moral analysis', in *Physician Assisted Suicide: Expanding the Debate*, M.P. Battin, Rosamond Rhodes, and Anita Silvers (eds). Routledge, New York and London, 182–202.

Gostin, L.: 1997, 'Deciding life and death in the courtroom', *Journal of the American Medical Association* 278, 1523–1528.

Holmes, R.L.: 2001, 'Is there a slippery slope from suicide, to assisted suicide, to consensual euthanasia?', this volume, 77–86.

Ikonomidis, S. and Singer, P.A.: 1999, 'Autonomy, liberalism and advanced care planning', *Journal of Medical Ethics* 25: 522–527.

Kamisar, Y.: 1998, 'On the meaning and impact of the physician-assisted suicide cases', *Minnesota Law Review* 82, 895–922.

Kant, I.: 1930, 'Lecture on Ethics', translated L. Infield, Methuen, London.

Kopelman, L.M.: 2001, 'Does physician-assisted suicide promote liberty and compassion?', this volume, 87–102.

Landman, W. A.: 2001, 'A proposal for legalizing assisted suicide and euthanasia in south africa', this volume, 203–225.

Levinson, S.: 1997, 'The court's death blow', *Nation* 265, 28–30.

Locke, J.: 1690, 'Second treatise on civil government', *Two Treatises of Government*, 6, 23, 135.

National Center for State Courts: 1993, *Guidelines for State Court Decision Making in Life-Sustaining Medical Treatment Cases*, West Publishing Co., St. Paul, Minn.

N.Y. Penal Law, Sec. 125.15 (McKinney, 1987).

N.Y. Public Health Law, Sec. 2989 (3) (McKinney 1994).

Nowak, J.E. and Rotundo, R.D.: 1995, *Constitutional Law, Fifth Edition*, West Publishing Company, St. Paul, Minn.

Oregon Death with Dignity Act, *Or. Rev. Stat.* secs. 127.00 et seq. (1995).

Planned Parenthood v. Casey, 505 U.S. 833 (1992).

Plyler v. Doe, 457 U.S. 202 (1982).

Povar, G.J.: 2001, 'Physician-assisted suicide – a clinician's perspective', this volume, 119–126.

In the Matter of Quinlan, 70 N.J. 10, 355 A.2d 647 (N.J. 1976).

Quill v. Koppell, 870 F. Supp. 78 (SDNY 1994).

Quill v. Koppell, 80 F. 3d 716 (2d Cir. 1996).

Quill T.E.: 1991, 'Death and dignity. A case of individualized decision making', *New England Journal of Medicine* 324, 691–694.

Resnik, D.M.: 2001, 'Physician-assisted suicide, the culture of medicine, and the undertreatment of pain', this volume, 127–148.

Singer, P.A. and Seigler, M.: 1990, 'Euthanasia – a critique', *The New England Journal of Medicine* 322, 1881–1883.

Tucker, K.L.: 1998, 'The death with dignity movement: protecting rights and expanding options after *Glucksberg* and *Quill*' *Minnesota Law Review*, 82, 923–938.

Vacco v. Quill, 117 S. Ct. 2293 (1997).

Washington v. Glucksberg, 117 S. Ct. 225 8 (1997).

Wash. Rev. Code 9A.36.060(1), 1994

Zoloth, L.: 2001, 'Job openings for moral philosophers in Oregon: physician-assisted suicide and the culture of romantic rescue', this volume, 103–116.

PART I

ON THE PERMISSIBILITY OF PHYSICIAN-ASSISTED SUICIDE

H. TRISTRAM ENGELHARDT, JR.

PHYSICIAN-ASSISTED SUICIDE AND EUTHANASIA: ANOTHER BATTLE IN THE CULTURE WARS

1. THE CULTURE WARS: AN INTRODUCTION

Protestations to the contrary notwithstanding, we do not share a common morality. Moreover, there are deep and divisive moral disagreements about medical matters. We are divided by substantive differences regarding the content of morality, even with respect to the meaning of morality. Is morality the reflection of a Platonic world of enduring values? Or, is it merely the product of evolution and culture, contingent and fraught with internal contradictions? Or is it properly an expression of God's will? Depending on the moral framework affirmed, physician-assisted suicide will be an element of patient empowerment or assisted self-murder. Physician-assisted suicide and voluntary active euthanasia[1] evoke controversies that reflect foundationally contrasting moral visions with important implications for bioethics and health care policy. To place the disputes regarding physician-assisted suicide in a larger context, this essay explores the depth of the moral disagreements that exist in secular bioethics.

Recent debates regarding health care reform illustrate the irresolvability by sound rational argument of fundamental moral controversies. At stake are incompatible understandings of justice and fairness. Some argue that justice requires equality of opportunity through redistributing property and forbidding the private purchase and sale of better basic health care. In contrast, some argue that justice requires respecting the rights of individuals to use their own resources for purchasing better basic health care, should they wish, even if the results undermine equality of opportunity. Some hold that justice requires taking from those who have in order to give to those who lack what is necessary for their basic life-plans, as well as in the service of equality forbidding the purchase of better basic care. Others hold that justice requires allowing individuals to use their own resources that are available after taxation to purchase from collaborating others better basic health care, as

Loretta M. Kopelman and Kenneth A. De Ville (eds.), Physician-Assisted Suicide, 29–41.
© 2001 *Kluwer Academic Publishers. Printed in Great Britain.*

well as luxury health care, despite the inequalities that might ensue. In short, some consider equality integral to human dignity and able to trump important liberty interests, while others recognize personal freedom as trumping considerations of equality.

The debates regarding the ordering of liberty and equality interests disclose different moral visions. Some recognize the guarantee of property rights and free collaboration to be core to human respect, despite consequent inequalities. Others in their reflections on equality discern a moral obligation of justice that brings into question the good fortune of those who have more opportunities, more wealth, and more resources for health care. Some in their reflections on equality claim an obligation to remedy if possible the unfortunate circumstances of those with limited access to health care, but without directly bringing into question the good fortune of those who are able to purchase better basic health care, as well as luxury health care. Some, in short, are moved by an egalitarianism of envy, others by an egalitarianism of altruism. Some regard inequalities of themselves evil, others regard inequalities evil only if they harm others. As a result, some would find injustice in some having better care than others, even if the others are not harmed and there is no likely system of distribution under which they could be better off (egalitarianism of envy). Others find inequalities to disclose the suffering of those who have less. The concern is then not directly about inequality, but about suffering (egalitarianism of altruism) (Engelhardt, 1996, pp. 384–387). The debates about justice, equality, and fairness reveal different understandings of the content and force of considerations of justice, fairness, and equality. In such circumstances, middle-level principles of justice underscore differences in moral vision rather than areas of accord. They show why there is disagreement, rather than common grounds for agreement about the proper allocation of health care resources.

The same point can be made in more general terms. Even if, *per impossible*, all were to agree that the goods of morality and social collaboration are those of liberty, equality, prosperity, and security, it is impossible to come to a principled agreement about the characteristics of a good society until one knows the proper ranking of such goods. Appeals to consequences, moral rationality, hypothetical choice theories, hypothetical contractor theories, etc., will always beg the question or engage an infinite regress. To discover or by sound rational argument to establish definitive conclusions, one must already have at least a thin theory of justice, the good, or values. Here there are fundamental disagreements (Engelhardt, 1996, Chapter 2).

Public policy developments regarding physician-assisted suicide and euthanasia promise a similar conflict of moral visions, this time with especially deep metaphysical and religious roots. The debates go very deep. They depend not just on different understandings of freedom, equality, justice, and ownership. The differences often turn on the meaning of the universe itself, the existence of God, as well as duties to God regarding one's own life and that of others. In the debates regarding physician-assisted suicide and euthanasia, one finds, as with abortion, that secular philosophical differences are more strident because they are joined with religious understandings that consider both as forms of murder and assisted murder. If anything, the conflict of moralities regarding physician-assisted suicide and euthanasia will be even more pervasive. Not all reproduce. Not all who reproduce find an occasion for abortion. However, everyone dies; there will likely be more occasions under which issues of physician-assisted suicide and euthanasia will come to the fore than with regard to abortion. Not all physicians are associated with human reproduction. Many more are associated with the dying and the death of patients. Hospitals can opt out of some of the challenges associated with abortion by not providing such services. Fewer hospitals will be able to avoid the challenge of dying patients. Physician-assisted suicide and euthanasia offer a foundational debate that will mark the future of bioethics.

These foundational disagreements raise a number of important moral and policy issues, three of which deserve special attention. First, to what extent do such disagreements bring into question claims regarding the existence of a common morality? Second, how do these disagreements press us to take moral diversity seriously? Third, what implications do such moral disagreement and diversity have for a secular state and its health care policy?

2. CULTURAL WARS:
WHY WE THOUGHT WE COULD AVOID THEM

First, in the shadow of the Second World War and in the light of new medical technologies, scientific advances, and with the challenge of new medical costs, many clamored for moral direction. Since nearly everyone recognized the horrors of National Socialist medical atrocities, the hope was that similar agreement could be secured regarding most substantive issues in bioethics. Few noticed that not only were the atrocities of National Socialism signally horrendous, they violated the core canons of secular morality as well as of most religious morality: the National Socialists were engaged in atrocities against individuals without their consent. At stake in these atrocities were fundamental forbearance rights such that there was no need to concur regarding the character of the good or the nature of human moral flourishing in order to recognize that a wrong had occurred.

In contrast, the allocation of scarce resources involves not just forbearance rights, but claim-rights against others. Abortion and physician-assisted suicide involve not just the forbearance rights of obvious moral agents, but also moral controversies whether, as in the case of abortion, fetuses are to be understood as having forbearance rights, and in the case of physician-assisted suicide, whether prudent choice and voluntary consent cure the major moral issues at stake. Although most will agree it is wrong to kill people against their wishes, there is no agreement about whether it is appropriate to kill at their request. The areas of moral controversy that plague bioethics do not for the most part turn on the fundamental issues that made the condemnation of National Socialist atrocities so obviously appropriate.

There are many reasons to avoid recognizing the full depth of the moral controversies defining contemporary bioethics. From the point of view of those who govern, it is in their interest to minimize moral differences and to claim that there is unanimity even in the face of underrecognized disagreement. Disagreement divides society. It is always possibly politically destabilizing. From the point of view of many engaged in moral philosophy, ethics, and bioethics, it also serves their interests to minimize, if not to deny, the existence of moral differences. If moral theorists are able to discover and articulate a content-full global ethics, then they will also be able to provide a unified general justification for governance. If the Enlightenment project of discovering by reason a content-full moral vision were successful, then:

(1) all would be disclosed as really being members of one moral community, superficial differences to the contrary notwithstanding;

(2) all would be bound by a content-full morality that could be rejected only at the risk of being found irrational;

(3) those who imposed a public policy elaborated in conformity with that morality would act with the authority of reason;

(4) those subjected to coercive force to conform to that policy should not find that force alien to their true moral selves, but rather restorative of their true, rational, autonomous behavior; and

(5) there would be jobs aplenty for bioethicists to elaborate the policy that should direct those who govern society.

(6) bioethicists would assume the role of secular priests: they would disclose the morality that should shape law and public policy as well as being able to serve as expert witnesses before court.

It is therefore in the interest of both those who govern and their bioethical collaborators to claim that:

(1) philosophers and bioethicists can by reason discover the canonical content-full morality, or

(2) philosophers and bioethicists can elaborate the common morality shared by all as humans, or

(3) philosophers and bioethicists can produce a moral consensus that can authoritatively guide those who govern, or some variation on one of these claims.

Bioethicists have strong interests in advancing a recapitulation of the Enlightenment project. Like the *philosophes* of the 18th century, they can hope to be engaged in fashioning an enlightened future, the French Revolution and the Reign of Terror to the contrary notwithstanding.

Bioethics has been further emboldened in announcing the existence of a single content-full morality by a circumstance reminiscent of the challenge from moral diversity that confronted post-Reformation Europe. In the 1950s, 60s, and early 70s, as physicians, biomedical scientists, and health care policy-makers clamored for direction, they were met with a cacophony of diverse religious responses. This circumstance was uncongenial for a number of reasons.

(1) The diversity of responses denied policy-makers unambiguous guidance.

(2) The diversity of responses disclosed a plurality of moral visions, threatening the unity of pluralist societies.

(3) America and Western Europe were becoming secular, making religious answers in principle uncongenial.

Secular bioethics then promised what the Enlightenment promised: a rationally defensible morality transcending religious differences and offering a unified moral vision.

The plausibility of this secular bioethical project was further bolstered by the success of commissions in framing bioethical principles and recommendations (NCPHSBBR, 1979). After all, if individuals with different theoretical commitments could agree to similar principles and endorse concrete health care recommendations, this should show that there is a common global ethic. Although at first blush this circumstance may appear to be evidence in favor of the existence of a common morality, an underlying consensus in society, or the ability to discover a rational moral fabric that should bind us all, closer consideration brings such a conclusion into question. If one is an adroit politician, one is unlikely to impanel a commission composed of individuals radically differing in their moral and ideological commitments from one's own or from each other. Feasible political coalitions are likely to be confused with an acceptable moral consensus that is likely to be confused with the canonical moral view. Though members of a commission may differ in the theories they use to reconstruct their ideological or moral commitments, those ideological and moral commitments themselves are likely to be fairly congruent. For such individuals, middle-level principles will in fact facilitate collaboration in the resolution of particular cases, the fashioning of guidelines, and the establishment of policy. In addition, the participants in such commissions are likely to experience the process as one of explicating or disclosing their common morality. There is much truth in this: they have indeed explored the morality they hold in common. This does not show that this is the only morality.

Imagine establishing a national bioethics commission to explore the morality of physician-assisted suicide with a membership that represents the actual range of American public opinion and moral commitments. Imagine also appointing persons with different moral viewpoints, such as Jesse Jackson, Jesse Helms, Mother Angelica, Bella Abzug, Thomas Quill, William Buckley.[2] One need only envisage representatives of groups both opposing and endorsing physician-assisted suicide and voluntary active euthanasia. When one has representatives of truly different moral perspectives, one can be confident that the debate will be intense and engaging, that consensus will not be reached, and that the use of middle-level principles will reveal differences rather than commonalties. The principle of beneficence, for example, will disclose differing views of the nature of the good, in this case, the nature of the good death.

The depth of the moral differences that divide us in morality in general and bioethics in particular is nevertheless often radically discounted and denied. This attempt to deny the existence of deep moral difference must in part be understood in terms of an ideology of consensus, a ruling false-consciousness, which serves the interests of political stability and the advancement of bioethics. Karl Marx and Friedrich Engels in *Die Deutsche Ideologie* give an account of how a false understanding of reality supports the ruling class. An ideology represents "the ruling ideas of the epoch ... The ruling ideas are nothing more than the ideal expression of the dominant material relationships, the dominant material relationships grasped as ideas; hence of the relationships which make the one class the ruling one, therefore the ideas of its dominance" (Marx and Engels, 1967, p. 39). This account suggests why the obvious may be so passionately denied: (1) obvious moral diversity is politically divisive and therefore politically destabilizing, and (2) there will be certain intellectuals, ethicists and bioethicists who can make a living supporting the reigning false consciousness, which in turn supports political stability. They serve as "conceptive ideologists, who make the perfecting of the illusion of the class about itself their chief source of livelihood" (Marx and Engels, 1967, p. 40).

3. PHYSICIAN-ASSISTED SUICIDE: ASSISTED SELF-MURDER VS. ASSISTED SELF DELIVERANCE

In the absence of a canonical moral vision that establishes a priority to life itself over other goods, or in the absence of a metaphysical understanding that establishes a duty to God not to take one's own life, it will not be possible to justify in principle the moral proscription of suicide, physician-assisted suicide, and physician-assisted euthanasia. As already indicated, such a canonical ranking of values cannot be established in general secular terms without begging the crucial question or engaging an infinite regress in the pursuit of a normative value perspective. Nor in general secular arguments will the invocation of duties to God be a clincher. As a consequence, disputes regarding a good death will be resolved among moral strangers by agreement and by not interfering with those who peaceably go their own ways. Since moral authority will be derived from permission, there will by default be moral zones of privacy, areas where one cannot enter save by permission (Engelhardt, 1996, pp. 68–74).

Insofar as one recognizes consent as core to the procedural morality binding moral strangers, the prime moral focus in physician-assisted suicide will be on the consent of those who participate, as well as on the costs and benefits of different policies. There will be an attention (1) to the authorization by moral agents of their own deaths, as well as (2) to the consequences of different policies for aiding and accomplishing voluntary killings. Under such circumstances, it will be impossible to establish secular moral barriers in principle to physician-assisted suicide and voluntary active euthanasia. Instead, the focus will fall on:

(1) the adequacy of the consent of those seeking assisted suicide,
(2) the absence of invalidating coercion,
(3) the presence of defeating duties to third parties,
(4) the possibility of untoward consequences, including the abuse of innocent parties as well as being prematurely dispatched, and
(5) the special effects of different policies on particular, historically conditioned understandings of the health care professions.

None of these considerations offers a bar in principle to secular bioethics, but rather raises various considerations to be addressed in determining how to establish moral rules or practices regarding physician-assisted suicide and other forms of consented-to killings.

Indeed, the secular moral burden of proof will fall on anyone who would coercively forbid physician-assisted suicide or voluntary active euthanasia. The ethos of death with dignity and the affirmation of rational self-determination makes death marked by suffering and lack of control profoundly unacceptable, especially in a society whose dominant culture values individual dignity and self-control. One should note that the focus is not on pain in such pleadings on behalf of physician-assisted suicide and voluntary active euthanasia. It is a loss of mastery over one's own life and destiny, which can be experienced as suffering. The argument in favor of suicide will, in such circumstances, not be blunted by adequate pain control or the availability of better analgesics. A death is unacceptable for many if (1) (a) it involves the indignity of the loss of control of bodily functions, (b) dependency on others, and/or (c) an inability to engage in that which gives one's life meaning when (2) there is the possibility of an earlier dignified death.

Here the affirmation of physician-assisted suicide draws on deep pagan roots which accord with Seneca's view that "Living is not the good, but living well." As Seneca argues, "The wise man therefore lives as long as he should, not as long as he can ... He will always think of life in terms of quality, not quantity ... [When] one death involves torture and the other is simple and easy, why not reach for the easier way? ... Must I want for the pangs of disease ... when I can stride through the midst of torment and shake my adversaries off?" (Seneca, 1958, pp. 202, 204–205). Considerations of the possibility of abuse will not in principle defeat such claims in favor of physician-assisted suicide. After all, those favoring physician-assisted suicide and euthanasia will need to balance the risk of being killed earlier than one would wish because of some abusive application of physician-assisted suicide policies with the risk of being forced to live longer than one would wish in the absence of physician-assisted suicide. If the first class of abuse (i.e., being killed prematurely) is likely to be much less frequent than the second (i.e., being forced to live longer than one wanted and thus suffer longer), and the second very highly disvalued, supporters of physician-assisted suicide will then be justified in moving to recognize physician-assisted suicide and voluntary active euthanasia as secular morally appropriate practices.

As the secular moral culture of the West becomes disconnected from traditional Western Christianity's proscription of directly intending the death of an innocent person, it will appear precious at best, if not perversely misguided, to draw distinctions between intention and foresight in the care of the dying. It will be a mystery to many, if not most, why one may engage in activities associated with an earlier death as long as one only foresees but does not intend the death of the person treated. It will be a puzzle as to why one may not also intend death. For example, it will appear morally meaningless to distinguish (1) those interventions that may without direct intention hasten death, as with the use of analgesics for patients who have demanded they be extubated, and (2) those interventions that with direct intention act to speed death when a patient has asked to be extubated. As behaviors, they may often be indistinguishable, with the only difference lying in the intentions of the agent. Such distinctions will simply not make moral sense to those no longer within a moral and metaphysical framework that recognizes the inappropriateness of directly intending the death of consenting individuals. For those who have been fully secularized and/or disengaged from Western Christian morals within which such concerns about intentions made sense, the distinction between (1) legitimate actions and omissions without direct intention of death and (2) interventions and omissions with the direct intention to bring about death will appear without moral substance, as was demonstrated in the opinions of the United States Court of Appeals for the Ninth Circuit on March 6, 1996, and the United States Court of Appeals for the Second Circuit on April 2, 1996 (*Compassion in Dying v. Washington*, 1996; *Washington v. Glucksberg*, 1997; *Quill v. Vacco*, 1996). Needless to say, the possibility of legal and cultural acceptance of physician-assisted suicide and euthanasia has generated a significant literature (Braun et al., 2001; Burt, 1997; Castro et al., 2000; Chevlen, 2000; Datlof, 1999; Emanuel et al., 2000; Gostin, 1997; Kamisar, 1998; Kavanaugh, 2000; Levinson, 1997; Rizzo, 2000; Sullivan et al., 2001; Tucker, 1998).

These changes notwithstanding, traditional Christians, Orthodox Jews, and others will still appreciate the moral wrongness of physician-assisted suicide and voluntary active euthanasia (Engelhardt, 2000, esp. ch. 6). This wrongness will be acknowledged within understandings at variance with the metaphysical, epistemological, and axiological commitments of a general secular morality. In particular, such will acknowledge duties to God not to take life, which duties are not defeated by concerns with suffering, dignity, or interest in self-control. Because of God-regarding obligations, physician-assisted suicide will be recognized by them as a grave moral evil. For bioethics and health care policy, this will have three major consequences.

- First, the debates regarding the propriety of physician-assisted suicide and euthanasia will remain. They will not go away.
- Second, strident disagreement will likely threaten the ideology of consensus and claims regarding a common morality.
- Third, and most importantly, such moral controversies may very well inspire the emergence of parallel, morally segmented systems of delivering health care.

This last point raises the prospect of a moral segmentation of health care delivery.

4. TOLERANCE AND CONFRONTATION

Although traditional Christians and Orthodox Jews should tolerate the involvement of others in physician-assisted suicide and voluntary active euthanasia in the sense of eschewing coercive interventions, tolerance does not require acceptance. Just as many find the condemnatory language of abortion as murder to be morally disruptive, so, too, the recognition and condemnation of physician-assisted suicide and voluntary active euthanasia as assisted murder and murder will be perceived on the one hand as morally disturbing and on the other hand as morally obligatory. As with abortion, so too with physician-assisted suicide, the judgment of the moral actions of those involved is likely to be forceful, substantive, and conflicting.

As with abortion, many will find it impossible to be moral collaborators. As a result, many physicians and institutions will likely not only refuse to provide physician-assisted suicide services and voluntary active euthanasia, they will also not refer for such services. One may even find some geographical areas without easily accessible providers offering physician-assisted suicide and voluntary active euthanasia, as currently is the case with abortion services. As a result, there will not only be moral controversies, but disputes engendered by the refusal to provide services that many will consider essential to a dignified death. On the one hand, the availability of physician-assisted suicide is likely inevitable. On the other hand, deep and persistent disagreements concerning physician-assisted suicide will likely lead to strong mutual moral condemnations and the refusal to provide such services.

5. TAKING MORAL DIVERSITY SERIOUSLY

One way to come to terms with the depth of these disagreements is to recognize and respect the integrity of moral diversity: to take moral diversity seriously. In health care, this may mean accepting the moral segmentation of health care delivery into provider groups committed to particular, content-rich moral understandings, many of which will be religiously informed. One might imagine, for example, a Vaticare health care system supported by the Roman Catholic church, but participated in by others who are opposed to abortion, to certain forms of third-party-assisted reproduction, as well as to physician-assisted suicide and euthanasia. One could even envisage circumstances under which a health care voucher system could develop, allowing people to pursue the realization of their own moral commitments within health care institutions and systems dedicated to their particular moral visions. This would provide structure for moral differences and even encourage a level of peaceable moral polarization. Such polarization, though, is probably unavoidable if one takes moral diversity seriously. The approach would avoid direct conflict.

Acceptance of moral diversity would require true tolerance on the part of those who preach tolerance: one would need to allow moral difference to have its place. Much today is said about the virtues of diversity. Societies, so it is held, are enriched by cultural and ethnic diversity. However, much of the praise for such diversity, though likely not disingenuous, is usually on behalf of a domesticated diversity without moral substance. It is a caged, tamed, and defanged moral diversity. It conceives of moral diversity somewhat on the model of a variety of ethnic restaurants with aesthetically pleasing variations on the project of being human. It is a human diversity that does not advance strong moral judgments or give rise to substantive moral disagreements. It is diversity on the model of a zoo where difference is caged. Yet, life, suffering, and death are serious matters. Our disagreements regarding life, death, and their significance will not evaporate. Medicine will often make these points of moral disagreement even more salient and unavoidable. Secular bioethics and health care will need to take this moral diversity seriously. The emerging acceptance of physician-assisted suicide and voluntary active euthanasia may support claims in favor of recognizing and coming to terms with this diversity.

Rice University, Baylor College of Medicine
Houston, Texas

NOTES

[1]   In this paper, assistance in suicide is explored under the rubric of physician-assisted suicide. However, there is no need for physicians necessarily to be involved. One could imagine a specially trained class of euthanatists able to assist in despatching people. What is probably desired by those seeking assisted suicide is a level of expertise that will deliver a prompt and painless death on demand. One could easily imagine this being provided by commercial euthanasia providers advertised in the Yellow Pages under such rubrics as "Kill Me Quick" and "Club Dead". For a study of Texas law, which until 1972 allowed suicide to be assisted by anyone wishing to be forthcoming, see Engelhardt and Michele Malloy, "Suicide and Assisting Suicide: A Critique of Legal Sanctions," *Southwestern Law Review* 36 (November 1982), 1003–1037.

[2]   I am in debt to Kevin Wm. Wildes, S.J., Ph.D. for our discussions concerning these matters and to his book (Wildes, 2000).

REFERENCES

Braun, K.L., Tanji, V.M., Heck, R.: 2001, 'Support for physician-assisted suicide: Exploring the impact of ethnicity and attitudes toward planning for death,' *Gerontologist* 41, 51–60.
Burt, R.: 1997, 'The Supreme Court speaks: Not assisted suicide but a right to palliative care,' *New England Journal of Medicine* 337, 1234–1236.
Castro, O., Gordeuk, V.R., Dawkins, F.: 2000, 'Caring for the dying – congressional mischief,' *New England Journal of Medicine* 337, 1049, discussion 1050.
Chevlen, E.: 2000, 'Caring for the dying – congressional mischief,' *New England Journal of Medicine* 342, 1049–1050.
Compassion in Dying v. Washington, 79 F.3d 790 (9th Cir. 1996), *rev'd sub nom.*
Datlof, S.B.: 1999, 'Beyond Washington v. Glucksberg: Oregon's Death with Dignity act,' *Journal of Law and Health* 14, 23–44.
Emanuel, E.J., Fairclough, D.L., Emanuel, L.L.: 2000, 'Attitudes and desires related to euthanasia and physician-assisted suicide among terminally ill patients and their caregivers,' *Journal of the American Medical Association* 284, 2460–2468.
Engelhardt, H.T., Jr.: 1996, *The Foundations of Bioethics*, 2nd ed., Oxford University Press, New York, New York.
Engelhardt, H.T., Jr.: 2000, *The Foundations of Christian Bioethics*, Swets & Zeitlinger, Lisse, The Netherlands.
Gostin, L.: 1997, 'Deciding life and death in the courtroom,' *Journal of the American Medical Association* 278, 1523–1528.
Kamisar, Y.: 1998, 'On the meaning and impact of the physician-assisted suicide cases,' *Minnesota Law Review* 82, 895-922.
Kavanaugh, J.: 2000, 'Wounded humanity and Catholic health care. Some contemporary thinkers have forgotten what "healing" really means,' *Health Progress* 81, 12–18.
Levinson, S.: 1997, 'The court's death blow,' *Nation* 265, 28–30.
National Commission for the Protection of Human Subjects of Biomedical and Behavioral Research (NCPHSBBR): 1978, *The Belmont Report*, [DHEW Publication (OS) 78-0012, 1978], Department of Health Education and Welfare, Washington, D.C.
Marx, K. and Engels, F.: 1967, *The German Ideology*, International Publishers, New York, New York.
Quill v. Vacco, 80 F.3d 716 (2d Cir. 1996), *rev'd*, 117 S. Ct. 2293 (1997).
Rizzo, R.F.: 2000, 'Physician-assisted suicide in the United States: Confronting legal and medical reasoning: Part two,' *Theoretical Medicine and Bioethics* 21, 291–304.
Seneca: 1958, 'On the sadness of life', in *The Stoic Philosophy of Seneca*, trans. Moses Hadas, Norton, New York, New York.
Sullivan, A.D., Hedberg, K. and Hopkins, D.: 2001, 'Legalized physician-assisted suicide in Oregon, 1998–2000,' *New England Journal of Medicine* 344, 605–607.
Tucker, K.L.: 1998, 'The Death with Dignity movement: Protecting rights and expanding options after *Glucksberg* and *Quill*,' *Minnesota Law Review* 82, 923–928.
Washington v. Glucksberg, 117 S. Ct. 2258 (1997).
Wildes, K. Wm., Jr.: 2000, Moral Acquaintances, University of Notre Dame Press, Notre Dame, Indiana.

REFUSALS/WITHDRAWALS AND
PHYSICIAN-ASSISTED SUICIDE

In *Euthanasia and Physician-Assisted Suicide*, Gerald Dworkin and I set
out a case in favor of physician-assisted suicide (PAS), and Sissela Bok a
case against it (Dworkin, Frey and Bok, 1998). The tactic that Dworkin
and I employ is to show that several important arguments in the arsenal of
those who oppose physician-assisted suicide do not work, and we seek
especially to explore and rebut arguments that purport to find a moral
asymmetry in intention and/or causality between refusal/withdrawal of
treatment and assisted dying. I want here to return and give more detailed
attention to an issue of causality in a particular kind of withdrawal case
that has come to figure prominently in discussions of physician-assisted
suicide, namely, cases of withdrawal of food and hydration.

An excellent discussion of the sort of case I have in mind can be found
in an article by Bernard Gert and others on "Patient Refusal of Hydration
and Nutrition: An Alternative to Physician-Assisted Suicide or Voluntary
Active Euthanasia" (Bernat, Gert and Mogielnicki, 1993). This title
expresses, in part, the view that withdrawing feeding tubes as a result of
patient refusal of (further) treatment is somehow quite different causally
and morally from physician-assisted suicide, a view increasingly heard in
contemporary discussions of causing death generally and of PAS in
particular. I want to challenge this view.

1.

I take the essence of opposition to physician-assisted suicide to amount to
the claim that a doctor may not permissibly supply the means of death to
a competent, informed patient who is terminally ill, who has voluntarily
requested the doctor's assistance in dying, and whose request has
survived depression therapy.

I am not here concerned with the deep split in the camp of those in
opposition to physician-assisted suicide who endorse this claim. One
group endorses this claim because of worries to do with whether the
patient is competent, whether he is fully informed in all respects,

Loretta M. Kopelman and Kenneth A. De Ville (eds.), Physician-Assisted Suicide, 43–57.
© 2001 *Kluwer Academic Publishers. Printed in Great Britain.*

including alternatives to physician-assisted suicide, whether his request is truly voluntary, and whether any such request does indeed survive depression therapy. Another group endorses the claim, however, *tout court*, for reasons to do with doctors causing death. For some who oppose physician-assisted suicide, the above sorts of worries, while perhaps present, do not in the end determine their view of the permissibility of physician-assisted suicide, since, even if by hypothesis no such worries are present, they still oppose physician-assisted suicide. Nor does the ubiquitous worry about slippery slopes determine permissibility either, since, even if by hypothesis we were to assume no such slope was in prospect, they still oppose physician-assisted suicide. Thus, some people oppose physician-assisted suicide precisely because they have worries of the above kind and in such a way that, were those worries to be removed, they could bring themselves to endorse physician-assisted suicide. To others, however, such worries are not the essence of the matter; even though such people often make very extensive use of them in their cases against physician-assisted suicide, such worries are not the ground of their complaint against physician-assisted suicide.

Nor is the claim on the mark that what is really at issue is that doctors may not kill their patients. In the physician-assisted suicide case with which I began, the doctor does not kill his patient; he simply supplies the patient with the means of death, which ensues as a result of the patient voluntarily using, say, the pill supplied. Of course, cramming the pill down the patient's throat would be objectionable, but nothing of this sort is at issue here. Presumably, then, what is forbidden is supplying the means of death to a competent, informed patient who voluntarily requests the pill with the aim of ending his own life, and it is obvious that those who oppose physician-assisted suicide because of worries to do, say, with slippery slopes need have no such view as this. As I say, I am not here concerned with this split, nor does it affect the discussion that follows. But it is important to notice it because, if the worries of one group could be removed, their core case for opposition to physician-assisted suicide disappears, whereas the other group would remain in opposition to physician-assisted suicide no matter what the state of these worries.

2.

What virtually all opponents of physician-assisted suicide insist, even as they insist that the doctor may not supply the pill, is that the doctor can withdraw food and hydration if, for example, the patient makes a valid refusal of (further) treatment. Not all withdrawal cases take this form, of course, since things other than food and hydration can be withdrawn from a patient's treatment; but it is cases of this form that pose a deep puzzle to those in favor of physician-assisted suicide, since it is hard to see what the morally relevant differences are between them and the pill case with which we began. What is the moral difference between the doctor supplying a pill that produces death and his withdrawing feeding tubes that produces death? How is one permissible, the other impermissible?

First, we need to distinguish between a case in which treatment has not begun and a case in which it has. In the former, if the patient asserts a (legal) right to refuse treatment and certain jurisdictions permit this, then the doctor honors the right by not beginning, by withholding treatment. With no treatment begun, the disease, illness, or condition of the patient is "permitted" or "allowed" to kill him. Insistence by the patient on such a right is, even though a number of doctors will not be happy as a result, treated in the media and by laymen as one way of committing suicide, of killing oneself. To say that one does not kill oneself, that the underlying disease, illness, or condition kills one, is treated by lay people, as best I can tell, as merely a way of speaking that lets others feel good. What matters is that insistence upon a right to refuse treatment, if the right is honored, leaves control over his life or death in the hands of the patient, so that, when the patient chooses death, death is what ensues.

From this, we need to distinguish a case in which treatment has begun, so that, when the patient now insists upon his right to refuse (further) treatment, the doctor can only honor the right by withdrawing treatment, in the withdrawal case at hand, by withdrawing food and hydration. The patient then dies of starvation. Here, again, is why having a right to refuse treatment matters: those who deny that a right to refuse treatment is the same thing as a right to commit suicide must nevertheless admit that such a right is the vehicle of suicide, where food and hydration is concerned. Withdrawal of food and hydration produces death, and the doctor withdraws the feeding tubes. The tubes do not come out as the result of accident, mistake, ignorance, or recklessness; they come out as the result of a deliberate act by the doctor.

There is no doubt about what ultimately ensues through the withdrawal of food and hydration: death. Notice, then, that such a case is unlike, say, certain ventilator cases, in which the doctor argues that he cannot be sure that the patient will die if the ventilator is removed. No doctor alive doubts the eventual outcome of the removal of food and hydration. Of course, it may be that the patient's underlying condition, as a matter of pure happenstance, produces death before the patient starves to death, but such an occurrence would be merely fortuitous. By withdrawing feeding tubes, the doctor must at the very least be prepared that starvation will overtake and kill his patient.

Of course, since the experience of the patient bearing the removal of feeding tubes (and undergoing loss of food and hydration) would be painful, a sedative is administered, and withdrawal takes place while the patient is under its effects. (This is sometimes popularly called "terminal sedation," but nothing in my paper turns upon any such way of describing the case, as something the doctor does.) I take it that, while the length of time in which the patient is kept alive after he asserts his right to refuse food and hydration can itself pose moral problems, it need not pose any special problem for our casual discussion here, where our ultimate concern is with whether, if the doctor honors the patient's refusal and withdraws feeding tubes, he is a part cause of the patient's death.

Second, our case is one in which the patient cannot see to the cessation of his own treatment but requires the assistance of the doctor – or of someone else. There is a moral issue here that I shall not bother to explore: how, if it is permissible for the doctor to withdraw feeding tubes and produce the death of the patient, can it be impermissible for someone else, say, the patient's wife to do the same? If the patient tells his wife that he insists upon his right to refuse treatment, and if his wife as a result removes the feeding tubes, what is there about her case that makes it impermissible but does not make the doctor's case impermissible? Notice that, whatever the answer, it cannot consist in two things. On the one hand, it cannot consist in the intention with which doctor and wife act, since both may act on the basis of morally admirable intentions, that is, to honor the patient's right to refuse treatment. On the other hand, it cannot consist merely in the fact that the doctor has the requisite knowledge for removing feeding tubes safely (and giving the required sedative), since non-doctors may possess this same knowledge. Notice further that the difference cannot consist in the probability that the doctor will not let extraneous facts influence his judgment whereas the wife might, since we have *ab initio* no reason either to suspect this in the wife's case or to dismiss it as present in the doctor's case. Possibly the difference may reside in the fact that the legal system recognizes doctors but not wives as agents of withdrawal, but that *does not in morality* appear to settle anything, as far as causing death is concerned.

Third, our case is one in which we may distinguish between law and morals. What doctors who support withdrawal of feeding tubes but not physician-assisted suicide want is that, in the former case, they are not held legally responsible for the patient's death; I take it also to be the case, however, that they want as well not to be held morally responsible for that death. There are cases where these things can come apart. For example, in some jurisdictions, there is no general legal duty of rescue, so that, in appropriate circumstances, even when rescue would pose no threat to the rescuer, one is not legally obliged to rescue, with the result that one is not legally responsible for the person's death. The person, say, drowned. But the fact that one could have saved the man, that a swimmer could have jumped into the water in non-threatening conditions to save a non-swimmer, does seem relevant to the question of whether one is morally responsible for the man's death. For if one could have jumped in but chose not to, then we have no reason *per se* to hold this fact irrelevant to the question of the moral responsibility for a death of the person who did not jump in. Every normative ethical theory I am familiar with, whether of a consequentialist or non-consequentialist strain, holds this fact to be relevant to one's moral responsibility. While the law in many instances allows people to ignore a drowning person, it is not obvious that morality permits this – or permits one to deny, *without argument and reasons*, moral responsibility for the drowning person's death. In our withdrawal case, what those who oppose physician-assisted suicide want is that the doctor be held neither to be legally nor morally responsible for the patient's death. Even if a particular jurisdiction were legally to permit withdrawal, indeed, even require withdrawal if the patient's refusal is a valid one (under the conditions I set out at the beginning), we have not thereby settled the moral issue. Appealing to one's legal position *ipso facto* does not justify one's moral position. Legally, you may walk past the non-swimmer; morally, most normative theories require more to be said than the mere fact that the law permitted you so to act. Legally, in a particular jurisdiction, it may be permissible for a doctor under specified circumstances to withdraw feeding tubes; morally, we have not thereby settled the issue of whether the doctor, if he acts or does not act, is partly morally responsible for the patient's death.

Nor can we be content to treat our withdrawal case as one in which, by his valid refusal of further treatment, the patient is regarded as the sole actor present, as if the doctor who withdraws feeding tubes were not there. The doctor is present and is the person who withdraws the tubes; death then, and then only, ensues. The patient's autonomous consent to what the doctor does as a result of the patient's valid refusal does not make the autonomous, voluntary decision by the patient to forego further treatment into the only morally relevant fact to the situation. (The autonomous, voluntary decision by someone to permit something violent to be done to themselves does not settle the issue of whether the one who inflicts the violence is morally responsible for what then befalls the person who so decided.)

The plain truth is that the doctor's withdrawal of feeding tubes is morally relevant to the patient's death. How? The answer is clear: the act of withdrawing feeding tubes helps cause the patient's death. So the only way I think a doctor can claim to be neither legally nor morally responsible for the patient's death in our withdrawal case is if he, the doctor, is not a cause, either wholly or partially, of the patient's death. The case cannot be reduced to claiming that the patient is killed by his underlying condition; for it is one in which, typically, starvation, not the patient's underlying condition, kills him. The patient is not "permitted" or "allowed" to die; the removal of feeding tubes causes his death by starvation.

Nor must we be deceived into thinking that the case should be construed thus: if the wife withdraws feeding tubes, the withdrawal causes death, whereas if the doctor withdraws feeding tubes, the withdrawal does not cause death. In either case, the cause of death is starvation through the removal of feeding tubes: what we go on to say morally about the characters of the wife and doctor may or may not differ, but we are not under any illusion that the removal of feeding tubes causes death by starvation in one case but not death by starvation in the other.

The approach, then, is to attempt to reach a conclusion about the moral responsibility for a death through a view about one's causal responsibility for that death. Two things need to be noted about such an approach. On the one hand, it is not an attempt to cast guilt upon the doctor: it is simply affirming that, in the way most moralities operate, what one causes to occur in the world is relevant to the issue of what one is morally responsible for. Indeed, we may, as a matter of fact, want the doctor to take seriously the autonomous, voluntary decision of his patient to refuse further treatment and may praise him if he does so; but the fact that we do not think he is of bad character does not settle the issue of whether withdrawing feeding tubes caused death by starvation. On the other hand, even if the law may treat the doctor differently from others, we would not have thereby settled the issue of whether in both cases withdrawal of feeding tubes caused the patient's death by starvation.

So what needs to be maintained, then, is that the doctor is neither a whole nor a part cause of the patient's death by starvation, when he withdraws feeding tubes. But then how can the wife be a whole or a part cause of a similar death in similar circumstances, if she withdraws feeding tubes? Of course, the answer might be that the law simply says that the one is not a cause and the other is, but, as I have been emphasizing, even if that is true, that does not settle the moral issue.

In other words, on the assumption that doctors who regard withdrawal of feeding tubes as permissible but physician-assisted suicide to be impermissible, the causal relation in which the withdrawal stands to death may be thought to be different from the causal relation in which the supply of the pill stands to death. But that differing causal relation, given that morality is in question, cannot consist in the claim that the law permits withdrawal, because that *per se* does not show that withdrawal does not cause death.

3.

As noted earlier, the withdrawal of food and hydration does not take place by accident, mistake, negligence, or recklessness. The doctor knows full well what he is doing and what the outcome of what he is doing will be. Not to know these things exposes the doctor to moral and professional complaints on other grounds. Of course, as also noted earlier, a doctor may be uncertain which will occur first upon withdrawal of feeding tubes, death by starvation or death, say, by kidney failure; but it is merely fortuitous whether or not kidney failure produces death first. What the doctor has certainly done, by withdrawing feeding tubes, is to enable the race between starvation and kidney failure as the cause of death to commence.

This last point cannot be stressed too much. For all too often in discussion of our type of withdrawal case there is the temptation, in order to remove the doctor from any causal role whatever in what befalls the patient, to argue *either* that the patient's underlying disease, illness, or condition kills the patient, which, if the patient starves to death, is simply false, *or* that the doctor, permitted legally to do what he does, *does not as a result* have a hand in causing death, which, equally, is false. Sometimes, to bring out this causal view of the matter, "but for" causation is appealed to: but for A having done x, y would not have occurred. But even that way of describing the matter does not actually capture the full causal point. For what requires stress is not that, but for the withdrawal of feeding tubes, the patient would not have died of starvation, though this is true; rather, it is that what enables starvation to enter the causal picture at all, what permits it to serve a causal role at all in the patient's death, is the act of the doctor in withdrawing feeding tubes. What appeal to the law and legality cannot remove is the fact that starvation is only able to overtake the patient and cause his death if the doctor acts one way as opposed to the other. And this is the crucial datum that enables morality to get a grip, namely, the causal precondition of the patient starving to death is the action of the doctor in withdrawing feeding tubes. Moreover, this is why the claim that the patient's underlying disease, illness, or condition killed him, besides being false when the patient starves to death, is radically misleading, since it makes it appear as if starvation somehow got in a position to cause the patient's death without any action by the doctor, and that is not the case. A vital part of the case is left out, if the doctor's act is not held to be part of what occurred, much as would be true in a case in which someone fell in front of the train, without it being added that someone pushed him. The train just did not kill the individual; rather, the individual was put into a position where the train could kill him, and how he got into that position, where being run over by a train could cause his death, is a part of the causal story of that individual's death. The same is true of the doctor's withdrawal of feeding tubes.

Moreover, our withdrawal case is not one of omission, which, if it were, might be taken by some to permit the doctor to argue, falsely, to my mind, that, since omissions are not causes, he is not even a part cause of his patient's death. Whether omissions are causes is too complex an issue to be tackled here, though I discuss it elsewhere (Dworkin, Frey, and Bok, 1998). In any event, our withdrawal case does not involve an omission. The doctor does not fail to do anything; he actually withdraws the feeding tubes from the patient's body. Action on the doctor's part can take the form, say, of giving an injection and thereby putting something into the patient's body, but it can also take the form of withdrawing feeding tubes and, therefore, taking something from the patient's body. The issue is whether the withdrawal of feeding tubes causes death, not whether the omission of something on the doctor's part causes death. In our case, he has not omitted to do something; precisely the problem is posed about the cause of death because he does do something. He removes feeding tubes. It is important not to be confused about this causal issue with regard to the issue of intention. Suppose we have two patients who have died of respiratory depression and two doctors who have injected largish doses of morphine into their respective patients. Suppose further that the intention of one doctor is to relieve his patient's suffering and the intention of the other is to get the bequest for his clinic that is part of the patient's will. In both cases, the cause of death is respiratory depression, which ensues as the result of the injection of morphine by the doctor. To be sure, one may want to go on to say of the second doctor that he is guilty not merely of causing the patient's death but also of murder. His intention, however, in injecting the morphine does not matter with regard to the question of whether the injection of morphine is a cause of death. The morphine, as it were, gets into a position to cause respiratory depression through injection by the doctor.

In ventilator cases, something similar is the case: the person who turned off the ventilator, doctor or wife, is a cause of death, regardless of their intention in turning it off. Again, the fact that we may want to go on to make other accusations against people who turn off ventilators does not affect this point. The patient is dead, in essence, because of inability to breathe. The person's turning off the ventilator enables the patient's difficulty in breathing to kill him; in turn, the doctor or wife enables this difficulty to kill him. Turning off the ventilator is a part cause of the patient's death, since the way the patient's difficulty in breathing gets into a position to kill the patient is by that act.

So it is in our withdrawal case: the patient only starves to death if feeding tubes are withdrawn, and the doctor withdraws the feeding tubes. His act of withdrawing the tubes is a cause of death. His intention in withdrawing them may be relevant to the further determination of additional things to say about his act, but that intention, whatever it is, does not affect the issue of whether the doctor's act of withdrawal of feeding tubes causes death by starvation.

But, it will be said once again of our case, the patient has consented to this withdrawal. True. But the patient's consent goes towards the issue of whether a moral (and legal) charge should be brought against the doctor for doing to the patient something that the patient refused to have done; it does not go to the issue of whether the withdrawal of feeding tubes causes death.

As I have made clear, if we can show that a particular act was a cause or part cause of death, then we can go on to invoke the view that causal responsibility for an outcome makes one liable to moral responsibility for an outcome in order to raise moral issues about the doctor's act of withdrawal. What is not true is what opponents to physician-assisted suicide want in this case, namely, that the doctor be held to be neither legally nor morally responsible for the patient's death because they want to hold that his act of withdrawing feeding tubes is not a cause of the patient's death. For starvation only gets into a position to kill the patient as a result of the feeding tubes being withdrawn. There is no difference between the withdrawal and lethal medication cases on this score: if the doctor withdraws feeding tubes, if he supplies the pill, he is a cause of death. To be sure, I agree that the patient's valid refusal of further treatment affects what we would go on to say morally about the doctor's act of withdrawing feeding tubes, but that does not show that that act of withdrawal was not a cause of death. With that causal relationship established, we cannot allow the doctor to deny all moral responsibility for the patient's death. Equally, I agree that the doctor's supply of the pill is a cause of death, and in physician-assisted suicide I agree that the doctor cannot deny all moral responsibility for the patient's death, even though a decision of the patient intervenes between supply of the pill and that death. But I am not here concerned with further things we might say about the doctor, morally: the claim has been by opponents of physician-assisted suicide that the withdrawal and pill cases are different causally, and I am suggesting that this is not the case. Withdrawal of feeding tubes is not an alternative to physician-assisted suicide, so far as causality is concerned. The doctor takes the essential step involved in enabling starvation to kill his patient. To say in the pill case that the doctor also takes an essential step in enabling his patient to kill himself does not show any causal difference between the withdrawal and pill cases.

4.

Again, it does no good to try to find a difference in intention between the doctors in the pill and withdrawal cases, so far as this causal issue is concerned. Nor, for that matter, need there be any difference. If the doctor supplies the pill, then even though a decision by the patient to take the pill intervenes between the supply of the pill and death, the doctor would in some sense seem prepared to see his patient dead; but if the doctor withdraws feeding tubes, equally he must in some sense be prepared to see his patient dead. The only way this could be false is if the doctor were incompetent, and did not realize what the result of withdrawing feeding tubes would be, or lucky, and the patient's underlying condition produced death before he starved to death.

Notice, too, something else about intention: in the pill case, it might be said that, in supplying the pill, the doctor must intend the patient's death, whereas in withdrawing feeding tubes, the doctor may well not intend this. Two points apply. First, in supplying the pill, the doctor may well not intend his patient's death; he may be supplying a means of death to a patient whom he suspects will not take the pill or who wants the pill for reassurance, if things get bad; whereas in the withdrawal case the doctor may very well intend his patient's death and see the withdrawal of feeding tubes as the means by which to bring this about. As I have said, in either case, the causal story, that the doctor's act is a part cause of death, remains true. Second, what the opponent of physician-assisted suicide has claimed is that doctors may not kill, not that they may not intend death. In physician-assisted suicide, *even if the doctor intends his patient's death* through supply of the pill, and he need not so intend, the pill can only kill the patient if the patient decides to take it; the doctor does not kill the patient. Loose talk of killing in this context, as found, for example, in Leon Kass's well-known article "Why Doctors Must Not Kill" (Kass, 1993; Gaylin, Kass, Pelligrino and Siegler, 1988; Pelligrino, 1992), simply muddies the water, since it mixes up causal issues with issues of intention.

Now I am not suggesting that there are not normative issues to be considered whenever we make claims about causality. Suppose a river is polluted and there are two causes, a major oil company and a very small manufacturing plant, and suppose we have no way of measuring the amount of waste either dumps into the river. If asked which is the more "important" cause, if asked which made the more "significant" contribution to pollution, then, if our aim is to find money with which to reclaim the river, it makes sense to find the major oil company more causally responsible for pollution, whereas if our aim is to deter even small polluters we may not want to isolate the major oil company in this way. On the one hand, the oil company has deeper pockets; on the other, we may fear other small plants will begin to dump their waste into the river, unless we make an example of this one. So there are clear instances where we find causal judgments encumbered with normative or valuational considerations. It is even true that we may judge a polluter not to be a polluter at all. Imagine the same case only now with a third party, a small boy who dumps a test tube of oil waste into the river: even though he did dump something into the river, and so strictly speaking is a polluter, we have no difficulty in understanding why we might judge his contribution to the outcome to have been so slight, as to enable him to get off the hook altogether. But in our withdrawal case, how can we judge the doctor's contribution to have been so slight as to remove him from moral responsibility for a death? Without his withdrawal of feeding tubes, the patient would not have starved to death, and our doctor knows this.

Well, it might be asked, what does it matter if I am correct in regarding the doctor as a cause of the patient's death in the withdrawal case, if I am also prepared to say that we want doctors to take seriously, whatever the state of the law, a patient's refusal of treatment? If I agree with all this and so with withdrawal of feeding tubes, what's the problem? The problem, obviously, is that withdrawal is posed as an alternative to physician-assisted suicide and active voluntary euthanasia, and the alternative is supposed to be grounded, ultimately, in differences in causal structure between withdrawal and physician-assisted suicide cases. I find no such difference. Moreover, though I cannot argue the point here, this absence of causal difference affects the entire mode of thinking that the distinction between killing and "permitting" or "allowing" to die is usually taken to manifest.

In our withdrawal case, what is wanted by those who see it as an alternative to physician-assisted suicide and active voluntary euthanasia, is that the doctor be seen as neither legally nor morally responsible for the patient's death. As I emphasized at the outset, merely to be legally free of imputation of a death is not sufficient; for the assumption, assuredly correct, is that no doctor would be content to be legally absolved of, but morally tainted by, causing a death. The only way this complete absolution can occur, I have suggested, is by holding that the doctor does not cause a death; for if he causes a death, he is at least *prima facie* morally responsible for a death. We may go on to let him off the moral hook, of course, but, from the point of view of contrast with physician-assisted suicide, the damage would have been done.

So we must probe carefully the argument, increasingly heard, that if the patient insists on their right to refuse further treatment and if the particular legal jurisdiction underwrites this right, then the doctor has no option but to withdraw feeding tubes. He has no choice; his hand is forced. He is helpless. Down this road can lie, though not in our withdrawal case, some very unpalatable issues that surface, periodically, when we encounter those who try to hide behind the law to shield themselves from moral responsibility for certain outcomes in the world. The claim that the law "permitted" or "enjoined" me to do this no longer carries the ring it used to, so far as moral taint is concerned. Such issues are not to the point here, however, since, in our withdrawal case, the death is not an accident, a mistake or the result of ignorance or negligence. It is knowingly and deliberately brought about. The doctor may see himself as forced to adhere to the law; but he cannot use this fact to elude causal responsibility for what ensues as the result of his deciding to go ahead with the withdrawal. For he could choose not to go ahead. It may be thought that this places the doctor between the devil and the deep blue sea: if he does not adhere to the patient's right to refuse further treatment, he may be legally liable, whereas if he adheres to the patient's right and withdraws feeding tubes he cannot avoid causal, and so perhaps moral, responsibility for the patient's death. This, I submit, is the case. What would then be at issue is whether we go on to ascribe (moral) guilt to the doctor, given the consent of the patient through his insistence on his right to refuse treatment. But in the lethal medication case we are in a similar situation, so far as consent goes: the doctor does not kill the patient but the patient, in full knowledge of the consequences, asks for and accepts a prescription of a pill that, if and only if he chooses to take it, will kill him, and he takes it. Consent does not separate the cases.

One final point: In our withdrawal case, if the doctor does not withdraw feeding tubes, then he fails to honor the patient's right to refuse treatment; but if he fails to provide the pill, there is no violation of the patient's right to refuse (further) treatment. A right to refuse treatment does not entail a right to be provided the means of death. So, why can we not say that this is the moral difference between our withdrawal case and our lethal medication case, since refusing to supply the pill does not violate the patient's rights, whereas not withdrawing the feeding tubes does?

For those who want to say this, however, there is a problem. It is obvious: as I have noted, a legal right to refuse (further) medical treatment is, if insisted upon, one way of committing suicide; taking the lethal pill, however, is another way of committing suicide. Why, if suicide itself is permissible, is one way of committing suicide, the doctor withdrawing feeding tubes, more acceptable than another way of committing suicide, the doctor supplying a pill that the patient then takes? Put differently, we need some reason to think that, if suicide itself is morally acceptable, the fact that a right to refuse treatment underpins our withdrawing but not our lethal pill case makes a conclusive moral difference in the cases of terminally ill patients. Otherwise, to say that a doctor may permissibly withdraw feeding tubes but not prescribe a pill because the former but not the latter is covered by a right to refuse treatment, is simply to place an artificial moral boundary on the manner of suicide. This claim is to pronounce some means of suicide more acceptable than others, without surveying all the moral principles that go into our judgment about acceptable means of suicide. For example, one principle increasingly cited in this regard is the merit of achieving a dignified end to life; and this lethal pill, as well as the withdrawal, brings this about. Another principle, increasingly cited, is that of the value of patient autonomy and a control over both life and death decisions that must be taken seriously by doctors; the lethal pill and the withdrawal achieve this as well. And so on. It seems merely arbitrary in the cases of terminally ill patients to say, given one thinks suicide is permissible in the first place, that having a doctor withdraw feeding tubes is acceptable but having him provide a pill is not, even though the patient sees both as means of committing suicide. Of course, if one is not prepared to allow suicide to be permissible at all, if, that is, one considers even suicide to be wrong, irrespective of the patient's autonomous, voluntary choice of suicide, then both the withdrawal and pill cases will have to be rejected, since both are, in the ways described, instances of means of committing suicide. In that eventuality, there is no moral difference between the withdrawal and pill cases, and the former cannot be used by way of contrast to the latter. So, the only way the example can even purport to work, is by suicide itself being held to be permissible, in which case we need arguments to show why the doctor withdrawing feeding tubes is more acceptable than the doctor supplying a pill and why some moral principle about a right to refuse treatment is more compelling than some moral principle about achieving a dignified end to life. Absent these arguments, I conclude that the cases are to be treated alike causally, without their being any other significant moral difference between them.

Bowling Green State University
Bowling Green, Ohio

REFERENCES

Bernat, J.L., Gert, B., and Mogielnicki, R.P.: 1993, 'Patient refusal of hydration and nutrition: An alternative to physician assisted suicide and voluntary active euthanasia', *Archives of Internal Medicine* 153, 2723–2727.

Dworkin, G., Frey, R.G., and Bok, S.: 1998, *Euthanasia and Physician-Assisted Suicide*, Cambridge University Press, Cambridge, Massachusetts.

Gaylin W., Kass L.R., Pelligrino E.: 1988, 'Doctors must not kill', *Journal of the American Medical Association* 259, 2139–2140.

Kass, L.R.: 1989, 'Neither for love nor money: Why doctors must not kill', *The Public Interest* 94, 25–47.

Pellegrino, E.: 1992, 'Doctors must not kill', *Journal of Clinical Ethics* 3, 95–102.

DAN W. BROCK

PHYSICIAN-ASSISTED SUICIDE
– THE WORRY ABOUT ABUSE[1]

In June 1997, the U.S. Supreme Court reversed decisions in the 9th (*Compassion*, 1996) and 2nd (Quill, 1996) Federal Circuit Courts of Appeal that had held that state laws prohibiting physician-assisted suicide (PAS) in Washington and New York, respectively, were unconstitutional (U.S. Supreme Court, 1997). The decisions left states free to craft policy on physician-assisted suicide and to prohibit it, as most states now do, or to permit it under one or another regulatory system, as Oregon now does (Oregon, 1995). While I believe there is a plausible constitutional argument that can be, and was, made for a constitutionally protected liberty interest in determining "the time and manner of one's death," as the 9th Federal Circuit Court's opinion put it, the present Supreme Court has made clear that it does not accept any such broad right. Some commentators, as well as more than one of the justices, have interpreted the Court's decision as leaving open the possibility of accepting a more narrowly framed right to physician-assisted suicide in the future, but for now the principal focus of efforts to secure such a right will return to the states, either through referenda or legislative action, where it had been before the two Circuit Court opinions.

There are several political and policy advantages to returning the issue to the public and to legislatures at the state level. First, any change in public policy to permit physician-assisted suicide will now occur much more gradually than it would have had the Supreme Court upheld one or both of the two Federal Circuit Court opinions and thereby struck down prohibition of physician-assisted suicide in all states. For what many citizens and health professionals see as a radical and dangerous change in public policy that threatens the well being and even the lives of many Americans, it is reasonable to use the "laboratory of the states," introducing the practice into one or a few states at a time. If the practice has bad consequences and unavoidable abuses as many of its opponents fear, a gradual introduction of the practice will limit their scope and enable the practice to be carefully studied and its abuses and harms identified. Possible changes in regulatory or other mechanisms that would

Loretta M. Kopelman and Kenneth A. De Ville (eds.), Physician-Assisted Suicide, 59–74.
© 2001 *Kluwer Academic Publishers. Printed in Great Britain.*

reduce those harms and abuses then can be identified, or instead, the prohibition of physician-assisted suicide can be restored.

Second, there is often a significant political cost in the Court's forcing a radical change on a highly divisive policy issue like physician-assisted suicide. While judicial review is clearly part of our overall democratic tradition, the Supreme Court is by intent the branch of government least subject to democratic control and accountability. When the Court forces radical change on such an issue, as it did for example with *Roe v. Wade* on abortion, its legitimacy to force such change is seriously questioned by many citizens (Roe, 1973). If the issue must be fought through legislative or referenda processes the result is more likely to be accepted as the will of the majority, and so to that extent legitimate, even by those who oppose the change. Moreover, since public opinion polls have consistently shown that a majority of Americans favor terminally ill patients having access to assistance in dying from their physicians, it should be possible to win these changes over time through democratic processes. This is not to say, of course, that the Courts should not protect unpopular or highly controversial constitutional rights of individuals – doing so is one of their central functions. Court review to uphold constitutional rights is intended to place a limit on democratic majorities and that is in part why I believe it should have upheld at least one of the two Federal Circuit Court decisions. My point is only that there can be a heavy political cost in its playing this role, as the continuing deep social and political divisions over abortion make clear. Moving more slowly through more democratic processes can reduce that political and social cost.

Third, had the Court found that outright prohibition of physician-assisted suicide was not constitutionally permissible, it would without doubt and correctly still have found that the states have a legitimate interest in regulating the practice. The result would have been litigation extending not just over years, but probably over decades, about what regulation is compatible with individuals' constitutional rights to physician-assisted suicide. Now well into the third decade since *Roe v. Wade*, such litigation is one reason why abortion remains such a prominent and divisive force in American politics. We have paid a heavy social and political cost for securing the right of women to safe and legal abortions. I should not be misunderstood on this point – in the case of abortion, that cost was clearly worth paying. In the case of physician-assisted suicide, where the right to refuse life-sustaining treatment effectively secures the right to determine the time and manner of one's death for most patients, the cost of not upholding a right to physician-assisted suicide is much less than the cost to women of not securing the right to abortion would have been. A calculus of the social costs of upholding constitutional rights is not, of course, the proper basis for deciding whether there are such rights – I mean only to note the lesser social and political costs of democratic legislation over judicial imposition on a deeply divisive issue of this sort. When the Court imposes a deeply controversial position, even when the position is supported by most citizens, one result can also be to undermine the legitimacy of the Court in the eyes of many citizens.

Fourth, if the right to physician-assisted suicide is a constitutionally protected right, it would be hard to restrict it to the class of persons to which even most of its supporters want to limit it. Most referenda and legislative proposals from supporters of physician-assisted suicide would limit it to terminally ill adults who are competent to make their own health care and other decisions. For decisions about life-sustaining treatment, the courts have consistently held since *Quinlan* that patients do not lose their rights when they become incompetent (*Quinlan*, 1976). Instead, surrogates, typically close family members, are entitled to decide for them exercising so-called "substituted judgment," that is, making the decision the patient would have made in the circumstances if the patient were competent (Buchanan and Brock, 1989). Moreover, many court decisions have made clear also that the right to refuse life support is not restricted to terminally ill patients, but is the right of all patients. If a constitutional right to physician-assisted suicide were grounded in the same fundamental rights and principles that ground the right to forego life support, it would be difficult if not impossible to restrict the right to competent, terminally ill patients. Moreover, the reasoning that would ground a constitutional right to physician-assisted suicide, such as that of either the 9th or 2nd Federal Circuit Courts, would likely support a right to voluntary active euthanasia (VAE) as well, on the grounds that to restrict the right to patients able to take the last physical action of using a lethal medication or other lethal process would impermissibly discriminate against patients unable to do so for themselves. But extending the right to physician-assisted suicide to patients who are not terminally ill and who are no longer competent, with decisions made either by advance directive or by a surrogate, and to voluntary active euthanasia as well as physician-assisted suicide, would greatly enlarge the potential class of patients who might receive physician-assisted suicide or voluntary active euthanasia and increase the risks that physician-assisted suicide or voluntary active euthanasia was not what the patient would have wanted. Such a broadened practice would unquestionably have greater potential for abuse and would probably not be supported by a majority of the public. If there is no constitutional right to physician-assisted suicide, however, the states can permissibly extend physician-assisted suicide to some persons, for example, terminally ill and competent adult patients, but not to others, in making reasonable policy judgments about the risks and benefits of different alternative practices and policies.

In the foreseeable future the debate about physician-assisted suicide will be principally a moral and policy, not a constitutional, debate and referenda or legislative efforts at the state level. This paper will address one issue that will be central in that debate – the potential for abuse of a legally permitted practice of physician-assisted suicide. This is probably the most serious concern of many, if not most, opponents of physician-assisted suicide, and it certainly played a substantial role in the reasoning of the majority opinion, as well as some of the concurring opinions, in the Supreme Court decisions about physician-assisted suicide. In some versions of this concern, it is the familiar slippery slope argument that proposals for legalizing physician-assisted suicide are only the first step in what would be an ever expanding practice of killing patients, a practice that would move far beyond justifiable bounds. There are both empirical and moral issues in the assessment of this argument against physician-assisted suicide. One empirical issue is the degree to which safeguards surrounding a practice of physician-assisted suicide would limit unjustified use of it. A second empirical issue is the likelihood that the practice would be unjustifiably expanded over time, for example as a result of a weakening respect for human life, to permit physician-assisted suicide in circumstances in which we now believe it would be wrong. A third empirical issue is whether the practice of physician-assisted suicide would be more likely to be abused than the currently accepted practice permitting forgoing of life support.

There are two central moral issues in the assessment of the potential for abuse. The first is which cases of physician-assisted suicide would be morally justified and which would be morally wrong and so count as abuses. The second is the degree of importance or seriousness of both the good and bad consequences of different public policies regarding physician-assisted suicide. All policy options regarding physician-assisted suicide and other forms of end-of-life decision making and care have both good and bad consequences, and so the evaluation of any policy option requires assessing the relative moral importance of both its good and bad consequences.

Needless to say, both these empirical and moral issues bearing on the potential for abuse of different policy options regarding physician-assisted suicide are uncertain and controversial. There are only very limited direct data on the first two empirical issues short of experience in the state of Oregon of the first year's operation of their practice permitting physician-assisted suicide provides no evidence of abuse (Chin, 1999). The only other related case from which inferences are often drawn regarding likely experience in the U.S. – the experience over the last decade or so in the Netherlands where physician-assisted suicide and voluntary active euthanasia, though not strictly legal, are legally tolerated under certain conditions – is itself highly controversial (VanDerMaas, 1996). The third empirical issue is difficult as well, despite the fact that a legally permissible practice of forgoing life support exists in the U.S., since there are no systematic studies of which I am aware that focus on abuses in decisions to forgo life support; abuses would be difficult to study in any event since they would generally be illegal behaviors for which there would be strong incentives to hide. Regarding the two moral issues, plainly there is widespread and deep moral disagreement both about which cases, if any, would be justified and which would constitute abuses, and, even more, about the relative moral importance or seriousness of the various good and bad consequences of different policy options. All this means that the objection to permitting physician-assisted suicide based on the potential for abuse cannot be decisively settled, but there are nevertheless strong reasons to be skeptical about it.

Consider first the fundamental, though rarely articulated, assumption underlying the potential for abuse objection to physician-assisted suicide. That assumption is that the practices with limited potential for abuse are the forgoing of life support, pain relief that hastens death, and perhaps, terminal sedation, whether the decisions are made by competent patients or the surrogates of incompetent patients; whereas the potential for abuse is much greater with physician-assisted suicide and even more, voluntary active euthanasia. As already noted, which cases count as abuses is itself controversial, but the importance widely accorded to informed consent and advance directives, at least in the case of forgoing life support, pain relief that hastens death, and terminal sedation, suggests wide agreement that decisions should follow the patient's wishes. Thus, decisions which conflict with what patients do, or would want, are abuses. The same standard is implicit in the potential abuses typically cited by opponents of physician-assisted suicide, which are subtle or non-subtle pressures for physician-assisted suicide that the patient does not, or would not, want. If this is the roughly correct standard for what constitute abuses, then even in the absence of data there is strong reason to believe that the common assumption about which practices are most subject to abuse is mistaken. Instead, the important distinction for the potential for abuse is between those practices in which the competent patient makes the decision for him- or herself and other practices in which the patient is incompetent and someone else must decide for the patient. A number of studies have documented that neither physicians nor family members can reliably predict patients' preferences regarding end-of-life care in the absence of explicit and specific discussion with the patient (Uhlmann, 1988; Tomlinson, 1990; Pearlman, 1992). Even when surrogate decision makers attempt only to determine what the patient would have wanted, they will often fail to do so correctly. Moreover, when surrogate decision makers have conflicts between their own interests or desires, or the interests or desires of others about whom they care, and those of the patient, we can expect further conflicts between their decisions and what the patients for whom they are acting would have wanted. This supports a strong presumption that the point at which the potential for abuse increases substantially in end-of-life-care decisions is when surrogate decision makers must decide for incompetent patients instead of competent patients deciding for themselves. And, of course, this means in turn that physician-assisted suicide (and even voluntary active euthanasia) are among the end-of-life decisions and practices *less* subject to abuse than are decisions by surrogates for incompetent patients to forgo life support, use pain relief that may hasten death, or employ terminal sedation. But are there other reasons for thinking that, despite this presumption, physician-assisted suicide would overall be more subject to abuse than these other widely accepted practices of surrogate decision making in end-of-life care?

One very important factor affecting the potential for abuse of any practice is what safeguards are erected to guard against the abuses most feared and likely. Proposals for model legislation to permit physician-assisted suicide, as well as the proposal that was adopted by referenda in the state of Oregon, typically have substantial safeguards (Baron, 1996). They include that the patient be:

–   An adult;
–   Diagnosed to be terminally ill (meaning likely to die within 6 months even with treatment);
–   Suffering from an unbearable and irreversible physical illness or condition;
–   Informed about his or her diagnosis, prognosis without treatment, possible treatment alternatives that might improve that prognosis, along with their risks and benefits (typically with a required evaluation of the patient by a second physician to confirm the diagnosis and prognosis, and documentation and witnessing of the discussion with the patient);
–   Offered other available alternatives, in particular hospice care and other palliative services, that might improve the patient's condition and change the desire for physician-assisted suicide;
–   Evaluated for competence by a qualified mental health professional, in particular to ensure that the patient's decision for physician-assisted suicide is not the result of treatable clinical depression;
–   Making an enduring (for example, with a waiting period of one or two weeks from the first request until the means for physician-assisted suicide are made available to the patient) and voluntary (free from undue influence) request for physician-assisted suicide;
–   Reported to regulatory authorities, in a manner that protects patient confidentiality while permitting oversight of the practice, as having requested and received physician-assisted suicide.

Now, of course, safeguards like these would not eliminate all potential for abuse of physician-assisted suicide – no set of safeguards could do that, and no practices in the real world are guaranteed to be free of all possible abuse. But the status quo in which physician-assisted suicide is generally illegal is not free of abuse either. One abuse of current public policy is that in all the states except Oregon that prohibit physician-assisted suicide it still occurs, but not openly and without any safeguards such as those above to control its practice. And if we compare the practices of forgoing life support, using pain medications that may hasten death, and terminal sedation, whether decisions are made by a competent patient or by a surrogate for an incompetent patient – in *no* state are *any* of the formal safeguards listed above in use, although all of these other practices, like physician-assisted suicide, also result in the death of the patient. This is further reason to believe that physician-assisted suicide would be less, not more, subject to abuse than these other widely accepted practices. Opponents of physician-assisted suicide, nevertheless, often point to the Netherlands, where there are a significant number of cases in which somewhat less restrictive safeguards are not fully adhered to, as evidence that these safeguards would be ineffective in the United States (Callahan and White, 1996). The opponents are correct that the safeguards would not be fully effective, but it is difficult to see why they would not at least reduce the potential for abuse with physician-assisted suicide below what it is now for these other practices that also result in death, but lack any comparable safeguards.

Opponents also argue that the potential for abuse would be greater with physician-assisted suicide than with forgoing life support and pain relief that may hasten death because many more people would be at risk of receiving physician-assisted suicide since it would not be restricted to patients receiving some form of life-support. But this is mistaken for at least two reasons. First, if physician-assisted suicide is restricted to the terminally ill, as it is in Oregon and in most of the proposals to legalize it, this would substantially limit those eligible for it and limit as well the amount of life that would be lost by any patient who did it; by contrast, patients can and do refuse life-sustaining treatment who are not terminally ill and who sometimes give up many years of possible life. It is difficult to know whether the potential pool of persons eligible for physician-assisted suicide would be larger or smaller than the pool of patients eligible to refuse life support. Second, and more important, we do know that in the Netherlands, where physician-assisted suicide and voluntary active euthanasia have been permitted for more than a decade, many times the number of patients die from withholding or withdrawing life-sustaining treatment and pain relief that hastens death than from physician-assisted suicide and voluntary active euthanasia. In the 1995 update of the original Remmelink study of 1990, it was estimated that 2.6% of all deaths were the result of physician-assisted suicide and voluntary active euthanasia (and another 0.7% were from ending of life without the patient's explicit request at the time at which life was ended), but 20.2% were from a decision to forgo treatment and another 19.1% were from the use of opioids in large doses (see VanDerMaas, 1996).

Are there, nevertheless, features of physician-assisted suicide that would make it more likely to be abused than decisions to forgo treatment or pain relief that hastens death? Opponents of physician-assisted suicide who focus on the potential for abuse typically cite several possible illegitimate motivations and incentives for physician-assisted suicide. First, with over 40 million Americans now without health insurance, many persons might choose physician-assisted suicide only because they cannot obtain adequate health care at the end of life. Second, even for patients with health insurance, there are well documented and widespread inadequacies in end-of-life care that could lead patients to choose physician-assisted suicide who would not do so if they had access to higher quality end-of-life care; the widespread failure to provide dying patients with adequate pain management and control is a special concern (SUPPORT, 1995). Moreover, the availability of the "easier out" of physician-assisted suicide might undermine society's and physicians' motivations to improve the care of dying patients. Third, dying patients are often difficult and demanding to care for, seen as the failures of medicine by many health care professionals, and emotionally draining on family members; moreover, many dying patients are frail, frightened, vulnerable and in a poor position to assert their needs and interests. If physician-assisted suicide is legalized, these factors could combine to lead to subtle manipulation or pressuring of some patients to choose physician-assisted suicide who would not really want it. Fourth, in an era of rapid growth of managed care in which cost containment dominates the health policy agenda, physician-assisted suicide may be seen as a money saving alternative to very expensive care of critically ill and dying patients, further pressuring such patients to choose physician-assisted suicide. Each of these concerns makes empirical claims for which data are scanty at best, yet the scope and probability of the feared effects are crucial to the weight they should be accorded; empirical research is at least as important as philosophical analysis in responding to them. Nevertheless, we can at least consider briefly whether there are more serious concerns about physician-assisted suicide than about forgoing of life support and pain relief that may hasten death.

The first two concerns, that patients without, and even with, health insurance will only seek physician-assisted suicide because they cannot obtain adequate end-of-life health care, are related. The safeguards proposed for physician-assisted suicide will provide some assurance that patients are informed about treatment and other alternatives, such as hospice care, but they will not always assure that those alternatives will be available and affordable. Some commentators have argued that the threat of physician-assisted suicide being permitted will lead, or already is leading, to strengthened efforts to improve end-of-life care so as to reduce the pressure to permit physician-assisted suicide, and to ensure that if it is permitted, few patients will choose it. However, we do know that even if physician-assisted suicide is permitted, only a very small proportion of dying patients will choose it. Consequently, we will still have to care for the vast majority of dying patients who do not choose it. All the reasons and motivations for professional and public concern to improve their care will remain in place. But there undoubtedly would be some patients who choose physician-assisted suicide who would not do so if better end-of-life care were available to them, just as there are now patients who forgo life support who would not do so if better end-of-life care were available to them. This is clearly a strong reason to improve the care of such patients, but is it also a strong reason to oppose permitting physician-assisted suicide, as many opponents suppose? I believe it is not.

Instead, our failure to provide high quality end-of-life care for all dying patients creates a cruel dilemma for public policy which should be recognized and acknowledged for what it is. Even if the many efforts now underway to improve the care of dying patients all prove immensely successful, there are two kinds of patients who will still prefer physician-assisted suicide. The first are patients who, even with optimal end-of-life care, will still prefer physician-assisted suicide because it best fits their view of a humane and dignified death; for these patients physician-assisted suicide is genuinely the best alternative mode of dying, and they constitute no policy reason for opposing physician-assisted suicide. The second kind of patient would not prefer physician-assisted suicide if they could get better end-of-life care, but since they cannot, they want physician-assisted suicide. What is the cruel dilemma that these patients pose for public policy? On the one hand, policy makers or individual physicians' reluctance to provide these patients with physician-assisted suicide is quite understandable, knowing that they would not want it if they could get better end-of-life care. On the other hand, we should be equally reluctant to deny them the physician-assisted suicide they want, and to make them endure a dying process they find worse than an earlier death by physician-assisted suicide, on the grounds that they would not want physician-assisted suicide if they could get better end-of-life care. To those patients, the prohibition of physician-assisted suicide in effect says this:

You cannot have the physician-assisted suicide that, in your circumstances, you quite reasonably want, but instead must endure a dying process that you find worse than an earlier death by physician-assisted suicide. Why? Because you would not want physician-assisted suicide if your care was further improved, although it will not be.

To those patients, that is indeed a cruel death sentence. The resolution of this dilemma is not simply to prohibit physician-assisted suicide, but both to galvanize efforts to improve the care of all dying patients *and* to make physician-assisted suicide available to those patients for whom physician-assisted suicide remains preferable to the best care available to them.

So the response to the first two concerns about abuse of physician-assisted suicide based on limits in access to health care generally, or to adequate end-of-life care in particular, is first, that these may as easily lead patients to forgo life support which they would not want if better end-of-life care were available and second, that this concern regarding physician-assisted suicide does not support prohibiting it, but rather both improving end-of life-care together with permitting physician-assisted suicide for those patients for whom it remains the better and preferred alternative.

The third and fourth concerns above are also related – they focus on the medical, emotional, and financial burdensomeness of critically ill and dying patients to their caretakers, families, and insurance plans, and the incentives these others may consequently have subtly, or even overtly, to manipulate or pressure them to accept physician-assisted suicide. Part of the answer to this concern lies in the safeguards noted above that are designed to ensure that requests for physician-assisted suicide are made without undue influence or pressure from others. Since these go well beyond any current safeguards for decisions to forgo treatment, it is hard to see why the burdens created by dying patients should not, if anything, more easily and frequently lead to undue influence or pressure on patients or surrogates of incompetent patients to forgo treatment than to choose physician-assisted suicide. And yet there are no data to my knowledge to support that involuntary choices to forgo life support are at all common, although they no doubt do sometimes occur. There is no well-documented problem of frail, fearful, and vulnerable patients now being pressured to accept earlier deaths than they wish, nor is there good reason to believe that this would occur with physician-assisted suicide if it were permitted.

Finally, the financial concern that physician-assisted suicide would be a cost-saving alternative to high-quality care of dying patients is not well-founded. A recent paper, co-authored by a strong opponent and a strong proponent of physician-assisted suicide, estimates the potential cost

savings possible from the introduction of physician-assisted suicide, and
concludes the savings would be negligible and insufficient to create
strong incentives, for example within managed care plans, to pressure
patients to accept physician-assisted suicide (Emanuel and Battin, 1998).

There is one last aspect of the fear of abuse objection to physician-
assisted suicide that I want to pursue briefly. This is a specifically
slippery slope worry that, although physician-assisted suicide would
initially be restricted, for example to competent, terminally ill adults with
safeguards like those noted above, the practice would soon be expanded
and loosened beyond control, to voluntary active euthanasia as well as
physician-assisted suicide, and to patients who are not terminally ill, to
children and the mentally ill, to incompetent patients either on the basis of
their advance directives or of surrogates choosing for them, and ending
finally with persons for whom there is no longer any pretense that
physician-assisted suicide or voluntary active euthanasia serve their
wishes, imitating the Nazi euthanasia program to rid society of "useless
eaters and burdens." Slippery slope worries of this sort represent different
kinds of worries about abuse than those I have been considering above
because they do not claim the specific practices of physician-assisted
suicide being proposed would be seriously abused. Instead, they are
commonly grounded in two sorts of claims: first, that the logic of the
arguments offered in support of the restricted practice of physician-
assisted suicide now proposed extends as well, and so would be applied
over time, to a much broader practice of killing; second, that introducing
even a restricted practice of physician-assisted suicide would erode over
time society's respect for human life so that we would come to accept an
ever expanding practice of killing.

Consider the first sort of claim, that the logic of the arguments of
supporters of physician-assisted suicide extends, for example, to non-
terminally ill and incompetent patients, and to voluntary active euthanasia
as well as physician-assisted suicide. Moreover, opponents of physician-
assisted suicide point out, in the case of rights of competent terminally ill
patients to refuse life support, those rights have in fact been extended in
this way to non-terminally ill patients and to decisions based on advance
directives or made by surrogates for incompetent patients, in each case in
important part because the logic of the initial arguments did apply more
broadly. I noted in the introduction to the paper that had the Supreme
Court upheld a constitutional right of terminally ill patients to physician-
assisted suicide, that right might well have been vulnerable to challenges

seeking to extend it in exactly these ways. But left as public policy decisions for the states to determine to whom and when, if at all, to make physician-assisted suicide available, states are free to make their own reasonable assessments of the benefits and risks of various extensions of physician-assisted suicide to broader classes of persons and/or to voluntary active euthanasia. Nevertheless, it is correct in my view that the fundamental moral principles and values that justify a restricted practice of physician-assisted suicide for competent, terminally ill adults do apply more broadly as this version of the slippery slope argument claims, and it is either a mistake or dishonest for supporters of physician-assisted suicide to deny that in the hopes of avoiding the broader controversies.

But it need be neither a mistake nor dishonest to limit the argument now, as I have done here, to the more restricted practice. Permitting only the more restricted practice would be quite reasonable social policy initially in order to gain evidence about the degree to which it can be adequately safeguarded and controlled. That evidence would be of fundamental importance in making any later policy judgments about the wisdom of extending the practice more broadly. There is a moral cost in restricting a practice of physician-assisted suicide to competent and terminally ill patients, and to permitting only physician-assisted suicide and not voluntary active euthanasia. There are equally compelling moral reasons for some non-terminally ill patients undergoing intolerable suffering, for some patients who have lost the capacity to make their own decisions but who clearly would have wanted actively to end their lives, and for some patients unable to perform the last physical action of ending their own lives, all to have access to a broader practice of physician-assisted suicide and to voluntary active euthanasia. The restricted practice of physician-assisted suicide that I have been concerned with in this paper would deny physician-assisted suicide and/or voluntary active euthanasia to some persons when, considering only their individual cases, there are compelling moral reasons to permit physician-assisted suicide and/or voluntary active euthanasia. But if physician-assisted suicide is extended to non-terminally ill patients, the seriousness and costs of abuses or mistakes increase, and if voluntary active euthanasia is permitted for incompetent patients based on their advance directives or on their surrogates' decisions, the risks of decisions that do not reflect the true wishes of the patient increase substantially. The potential risks of increased seriousness and frequency of abuse from these extensions or expansions of physician-assisted suicide may or may not be too great to warrant doing so. But even if the logic of the argument for the restricted practice of physician-assisted suicide does extend more broadly, it is not unreasonable caution to wait until we have experience with the more restricted practice before we decide which, if any, additional steps we wish to take on the slope.

The other version of the slippery slope worry is that any practice of actively taking life, such as physician-assisted suicide, will inevitably erode respect for human life, and set us on a path towards ever wider killing. Only time and experience with a practice of physician-assisted suicide could decisively refute this concern, but the fundamental role of individual self-determination or autonomy in the broad social movement over the last several decades in the United States to secure for patients control over their dying is a formidable bulwark against movement down that feared path. Respecting the self-determination of individual human beings in no way supports practices that would take the lives of persons against their wishes.

As I stated at the outset of this section, there is no denying the presence of widespread concern that physician-assisted suicide would be subject to much greater abuse than are the currently accepted practices of forgoing life support, pain relief that can hasten death, and terminal sedation. I have suggested a number of reasons, however, why I believe that concern is not well founded. Indeed, I would reiterate that abuse and mistake are more likely in practices in which surrogates make decisions for incompetent patients, and so concern to prevent abuse by erecting safeguards to protect patients might better focus there than on physician-assisted suicide.

CONCLUSION

I have not attempted in this paper to develop what I see as the main positive moral argument in support of physician-assisted suicide. I have argued elsewhere that the moral grounds that undergird the consensus about patients' rights to decide about life support can support physician-assisted suicide in at least some cases; many, perhaps even most, opponents of physician-assisted suicide do not deny that (Brock, 1992; Brock, 1996). Nor have I pursued the fundamental moral issues in a general account of why and when taking human life is morally wrong, although these issues certainly account for some of the disagreement about physician-assisted suicide.

Instead, I have focused on what I believe is one of the most common and influential arguments against changing public policy to permit physician-assisted suicide, an argument made by many who grant that some individual cases of physician-assisted suicide are morally justified – a legalized practice of physician-assisted suicide would be subject to intolerable abuse. I have argued that it is when someone else must make end-of-life decisions for incompetent patients, as compared with decisions made by competent patients themselves, that the potential for abuse increases substantially, and this suggests that physician-assisted suicide (and voluntary active euthanasia) is less, not more, subject to abuse than surrogate decisions for incompetent patients to forgo life support, to employ pain medications that risk hastening death, or to employ terminal sedation. Yet virtually no one argues, nor is there any evidence, that these forms of surrogate decision making are being intolerably abused. Moreover, I have offered several additional reasons to believe that physician-assisted suicide has less potential for abuse than other forms of end-of-life decisions and care. The worry about abuse of physician-assisted suicide has been widely influential in the moral, legal, and policy debate over physician-assisted suicide, but it is in my view unpersuasive. Progress in changing public policy to permit physician-assisted suicide depends, at this point in time, at least as much on undermining this, and other common objections to physician-assisted suicide, as it does on reiterating the familiar moral case in support of it.

Brown University
Providence, Rhode Island

NOTE

[1]   This paper is drawn from my longer paper, 'A Critique of Three Objections to Physician Assisted Suicide,' *Ethics*, 109 (1999) 519–547, and is reprinted here with permission of the University of Chicago Press.

REFERENCES

Baron, C.H. et al.: 1996, 'A model state statute to authorize and regulate physician-assisted suicide', *Harvard Journal of Legislation* 331, 1–34.

Brock, D.W.: 1985, 'Taking human life', *Ethics* 95, 851–865.

Brock, D.W.: 1992, 'Voluntary active euthanasia', *Hastings Center Report* 22, 10–22.

Brock, D.W.: 1996, 'Death and dying', in *Medical Ethics 2nd Ed.* ed. R. Veatch, Jones and Bartlett, Boston.

Buchanan, A. E. and Brock, D. W.: 1989, *Deciding for Others: The Ethics of Surrogate Decision Making*, Cambridge University Press, Cambridge.

Callahan, D. and White, M.: 1996, 'The legalization of physician-assisted suicide: creating a regulatory potemkin village', *University of Richmond Law Review* 30, 1–83.

Chin, A.E.: 1999, 'Legalizing physician-assisted suicide in Oregon – the first year's experience', *The New England Journal of Medicine* 340, 577–583.

Compassion in Dying v. Washington, 79 F3d 790 (9th Cir 1996) (en banc).

Emanuel, E.J. and Battin, M.: 1998, 'What are the potential cost savings from legalizing physician-assisted suicide?', *The New England Journal of Medicine* 339, 167–172.

Oregon Death with Dignity Act, Or. Rev. Stat. 127. 800–827 (1995).

Pearlman, R.A. et al.: 1992, 'Spousal understanding of patient quality of life: implications for surrogate decisions', *Journal of Clinical Ethics* 3,2, 114–121.

Quill v. Vacco, 80 F3d 716 (2d Cir 1996).

In re Quinlan, 355 A2d 647 (NJ), *cert denied* 429 US 922 (1976).

Roe v. Wade, 410 U.S. 113 (1973).

The SUPPORT Principal Investigators for the SUPPORT Project, 1995, 'A controlled trial to improve care for seriously ill hospitalized patients: the study to understand prognoses and preferences for outcomes and risks of treatment,' *Journal of the American Medical Association* 274, 1591–1598.

Tomlinson, T. et al.: 1990, 'An empirical study of proxy consent for elderly persons', *Gerontologist* 30, 54–61.

U.S. Supreme Court, 117 SCT 2258 (1997) and 117 SCT 2293 (1997).

Uhlmann, R.F. et al.: 1988, 'Physicians' and spouses' predictions of elderly patients' treatment preferences', *Journal of Gerontology* 43, 115–121.

VanDerMaas, P.F. et al.: 1996, 'Euthanasia, physician-assisted suicide, and other medical practices involving the end of life in The Netherlands, 1990–95', The *New England Journal of Medicine* 335, 1699–1705.

PART II

CHALLENGING THE CASE FOR
PHYSICIAN-ASSISTED SUICIDE

ROBERT L. HOLMES

IS THERE A SLIPPERY SLOPE FROM SUICIDE, TO ASSISTED SUICIDE, TO CONSENSUAL EUTHANASIA?

In the Supreme Court decisions (*Washington v. Glucksberg* and *Vacco v. Quill*, 1997), Chief Justice Rehnquist wrote that "opposition to and condemnation of suicide and, therefore, of assisting suicide are consistent and enduring themes of our philosophical, legal, and cultural heritages." While one might question this with regard to our philosophical heritage, Rehnquist is certainly right in the implied judgment that opposition to suicide is *ipso facto* opposition to assisted suicide. What I want to consider is the other side of the coin. I want to consider whether *acceptance* of suicide commits one to acceptance of assisted suicide (AS).[1] Further, I want to consider whether acceptance of AS commits one to acceptance of euthanasia (EU).[2] For many fear there is a slippery slope here. They fear that if assisted suicide becomes acceptable, society will be led inexorably to accept euthanasia as well. To those who oppose euthanasia, that would be a bad thing. To those who support euthanasia it would be a good thing. But whether or not both sides can be brought into agreement on that issue, they should, in principle, be able to agree on whether there is a slippery slope here.[3]

A word is in order about what one might mean by a slippery slope. One might mean that, whatever the moral and legal considerations on one side or the other, acceptance of assisted suicide would in fact lead eventually to the acceptance of euthanasia. Whether there is a slippery slope in this sense is essentially a factual question. As important as it is (and from a purely practical standpoint it is among the most important policy questions), it does not raise any central philosophical issues.[4] But one might mean that there are logical and perhaps moral reasons why, if suicide is generally accepted, assisted suicide and euthanasia should be accepted as well – whether or not they are likely to be. Clearly, there might be a slippery slope in the first sense without there being one in the second sense, and vice-versa. People might, as a matter of fact, come to accept assisted suicide and euthanasia if suicide were commonly accepted without there being any compelling logical or moral reasons to do so. By the same token, there might be overriding logical and moral reasons why people should accept assisted suicide and euthanasia even if they do not.

Loretta M. Kopelman and Kenneth A. De Ville (eds.), Physician-Assisted Suicide, 77–86.
© 2001 *Kluwer Academic Publishers. Printed in Great Britain.*

It is the second of these senses that interests me. It raises important philosophical questions. Does *consistency* require that if one accepts suicide, one must accept assisted suicide and euthanasia as well? Or are there morally relevant dissimilarities among the three such that one can quite consistently regard suicide as morally permissible but deny – or at least question – the permissibility of the other two? I shall argue that there are such dissimilarities. If this is correct, then whether or not there is a slippery slope in the first sense, there is none in the second.

1.

Let us begin by considering a line of reasoning that might be thought to lead us down the slope in question.

A.1.   One may permissibly take one's own life.[5]

  2.   Whatever one may permissibly do, one may permissibly request another's assistance in doing.

Therefore:

  3.   One may permissibly request another's assistance in taking one's own life.

  4.   Whatever one may permissibly request another's assistance in doing, one may permissibly request another to do on one's behalf.

Therefore:

  5.   One may permissibly request another to take one's own life.

Despite the argument's initial plausibility, premise (2) is suspect. There are things that are permissible for me to do but impermissible for me to request another's assistance in doing. If my elderly neighbor gives me permission to pick apples from her tree, that does not make it right for me to ask your help in picking them. The permission was for *me* to pick them. If she is wary of people but trusting of me, the intrusion of another person may be unintended, unexpected, and unwanted. Similarly, there are many acts of intimacy that are permissible with a spouse or lover but for which it would be wrong to request someone's assistance in performing.

It might be objected, of course, that premise (2) refers only to what I may permissibly *request* another's assistance in doing. It does not say that the other would be justified in complying with the request. So – it might be argued – these considerations do not suffice to show that (2) is false.

This objection might seem to be a mere quibble, but there is a point to it. If we assume that it really is only requests that are being talked about in (2)–(5) – with no implication regarding compliance – then a case could be made for considering the argument sound as well as valid. But understood in this way, the argument fails for other reasons. For its merely being permissible for me to *request* your assistance in committing suicide does not suffice to show that AS is permissible. Nor does the permissibility of my requesting that you euthanize me show that EU is permissible. The permissibility of AS and EU (unlike that of suicide) presupposes the permissibility of the acts of *both* the primary agent (the one whose suicide or euthanization is at issue) and the secondary agent (the one assisting the suicide or performing the euthanasia). The argument, even if assumed to be sound, at best establishes the permissibility of only one component of the justification of assisted suicide and euthanasia. This is a conceptual point regarding the meanings of assisted suicide and consensual euthanasia.

So let us modify the argument to strengthen the premise (3) and the conclusion, (5), so that if they can be established, they would suffice to establish the permissibility of AS and EU.

B. 1.   One may permissibly take one's own life.
   2.   Whatever one may permissibly do one may request another's assistance in doing.

Therefore:

   3.   One may permissibly enlist another's assistance in taking one's own life.
   4.   Whatever one may permissibly enlist another's assistance in doing one may permissibly authorize another to do on one's behalf.

Therefore:

   1.   One may permissibly authorize another to take one's own life.

But this remedy comes at a cost. For while argument A is arguably both valid and sound on our present understanding of it, argument B is not valid. It contains a non sequitur in the transition from (2) to (3). By making explicit the gap between one person's *requesting* assistance in suicide and another's *complying* with that request, the argument now reveals the necessity of bridging that gap. The mere fact that it may be permissible for one person to do something does not suffice to make it permissible for anyone else to assist him in doing it (we are assuming now that the permissibility of A's enlisting B's assistance in doing something implies the permissibility of B's providing that assistance). Nonetheless, in the sorts of contexts that realistically could be expected to be most common with regard to AS (where it is widely – and perhaps unjustifiably – assumed that the assistance would come from a physician), there is some plausibility to supposing that the permissibility of suicide would extend at least to the permissibility of enlisting a physician's aid in the act. So let us provisionally accept (2) and (3). We shall later consider other reasons for rejecting them.

Let us look then more closely at (4), which bears the burden of warranting the transition from (3) to (5). May I authorize someone to do anything I may permissibly enlist that person's assistance in doing myself?[6]

There is a way of thinking in social and political thought that would seem to support saying that I can. It relies heavily on an assumed transferability of moral authorizations. In the spirit of Hobbes and Locke, it holds that if I have a right, I may, in appropriate circumstances, transfer that right to someone (or something) else. Since rights entail permissions, if one may transfer rights, one may transfer at least some permissions. Robert Nozick's argument for the justification of the state, for example, proceeds in this way. It relies on the claim that individuals have a right of self-defense and may transfer that right to others (in protective agencies) to exercise on their behalf. Through this process there eventually arises – without any violation of rights – a dominant protective agency with a monopoly of power, that is, a rudimentary state (Nozick, 1974, Part I). Michael Walzer does much the same in justifying war, arguing that states have the right to make war simply as the collectivization of the right of individuals to self-defense (Walzer, 1977, p. 54).

But however venerable that tradition, I think this transition cannot be made. Even if we provisionally accept (3) it seems clear that (3) and (4) do not suffice to establish (5). The reason they do not is that (4) is false, or at the very least, highly suspect. We cannot always permissibly authorize others to do for us things they may assist us in doing ourselves. If I am a brain surgeon and you are a certified nurse, I may enlist your assistance in surgery, but I may not permissibly authorize you to perform the surgery for me. Likewise, if I owe a debt of gratitude, I may enlist another's assistance in discharging that debt. But it will not do – at least will not always do – for me to authorize that other to do for me the act which, if I were to do it, would constitute discharging the debt. Bound up in the notion of a duty of gratitude is the idea that it is something that *I owe*. It requires not just the production of a certain outcome but the production of that outcome by me.[7] And if I have wrongfully harmed you, it is arguably incumbent upon *me* to make good to you the harm that I have done, not merely to see that it is rectified. The whole idea behind restorative justice is that the offender must *personally* remedy the wrong he has done; it is not enough to send another to restore, repair, or replace what he has stolen or damaged of yours, or to send apologies through a messenger. I may ask your help in doing the dishes, shoveling the driveway, or changing a tire, and if I am lucky I may even get you to do these things for me. What matters in these cases is that the dishes get done, the driveway cleared, and the tire changed; the means by which they get done are not usually important. But duties of gratitude and reparation require not only that certain ends be achieved, but that they be achieved by certain *means* – through the personal commitment and effort of the one having the obligation.

2.

A more serious objection is that the argument we have been considering tries to establish too much, that premise (2) rather than asserting that whatever one may permissibly do one may permissibly request another's assistance in doing, need assert only that whatever one may permissibly do *to oneself* one may permissibly request another's assistance in doing. This, after all, fits more closely the case of assisted suicide, since it is part of the meaning of suicide – assisted or not – that it is an instance of killing yourself, and killing yourself is surely a paradigm case of doing something to yourself.[8] Premise (4) could likewise be altered, *mutatis mutandis*. At the same time, we might modify (2) so as to eliminate the non sequitur in B. By recasting (2) to state that whatever we may permissibly do to ourselves we may permissibly enlist another's aid in doing – where that is understood to imply that the other is justified in providing the assistance – the argument becomes valid. With these changes we get a closely related but distinguishable argument:

C. 1.   One may permissibly take one's own life.
   2.   Whatever one may permissibly do to oneself one may permissibly enlist another's assistance in doing.
Therefore:

3.   One may permissibly enlist another's assistance in taking one's own life.

4.   Whatever one may permissibly enlist another's assistance in doing to oneself, one may authorize another to do on one's behalf.

Therefore:

1.   One may permissibly authorize another to take one's own life.

Recall that we have been provisionally accepting (2) and (3). Since (3) now follows logically from (1) and (2), and we are not for purposes of the present discussion questioning (1), whether (3) is true depends upon whether (2) is true. But even recast in this way (2) still runs afoul of the same consideration affecting the transition from A (2) to A (3). In (1) all that is at stake is the permissibility of the performance of an act by the primary agent. But in (2) and (3) as well as in (4) and (5) the act of another person is centrally involved. In (3) it is the act of assisting another in killing himself. In (5) it is killing another person. Clearly, the act of requesting another to help you kill yourself is a different act from that of complying with that request. Moreover, the act of authorizing another to kill you on your behalf is a different act from the act of killing so authorized. Finally, killing another person is a different act – and arguably a different *kind* of act – from killing yourself or enlisting help in killing yourself or authorizing someone to kill you on your behalf. So the problem of bridging the gap between the permissibility of what the primary agent may do and the permissibility of what the secondary agent may do persists. Only now rather than being explicit in the structure of the argument (accounting for the invalidity of B), it is concealed in premises (2) and (4). This, I shall argue, makes (2) and (4) false, and the argument, though valid, unsound.

I have thus far emphasized moral considerations that relate to the primary agent and which serve as moral requirements in his or her discharge of obligations. What about on the side of the secondary agent? Are there moral considerations there which likewise impede any simple transition from what the primary agent may do to what the secondary agent may do?

Arguably, it is part of the very idea of morality that every act (meaning every free, uncoerced, voluntary act) is susceptible of moral assessment. Every act, in other words, is either right or wrong, and if right, is either merely permissible or obligatory. It is not that every act need in fact to be so assessed, only that it is relevant always to ask for such an assessment.

It is always relevant whether what we propose to do is right, and if so, for what reasons.

Now the mere fact that I may be morally justified in consenting to your killing me (as (5) establishes), or in authorizing your so doing to whatever extent I am entitled to, does not *in and of itself* suffice to establish that it is right for you to kill me. My authorizing you is one act (which, *ex hypothesi*, we are assuming to be permissible); your killing me is another. And that act is susceptible of moral assessment on its own. The fact that I have consented to your doing something to me, or authorized you to do it, or even ordered you to do it, does not, *in and of itself*, entail that it is morally permissible for you *to do* it. Once it is recognized that these are two acts, the possibility must be acknowledged that they may sometimes have radically different consequences. One consequence of your complying with my request or authorization is my death. It is not a consequence of the request alone or the authorization alone. Another consequence might be your arrest and conviction for homicide. That is not a consequence of what I do. A third might be that, justifiably or not, you might come to feel enormous guilt for having dispatched me, take to strong drink, and fall hopelessly into ruin. With a little imagination, one could likewise hypothesize equally felicitous consequences that would ensue from the one act and not from the other. This suggests that the moral evaluation of the two acts might differ radically on any view of morality that weighs heavily the consequences of individual acts in the determination of right and wrong.

But the evaluations might differ on non-consequentialist moral theories as well. The further determination of the rightness or wrongness of your compliance with my request or authorization – even if the request or authorization is itself considered permissible – cannot be made in the absence of any consideration of your circumstances and other obligations, commitments, and responsibilities you may have, that is, in independence of the broader context in which the contemplated act might take place. If nothing else, legal constraints, while not decisive, are always morally relevant considerations. And if, as is true in this and most countries today, that euthanasia is prohibited, then that is a relevant – though again not decisive – moral consideration. Or if you should have deeply-rooted religious objections to killing another human being, that, too, is a relevant consideration. As would be any prohibitions contained in the professional ethics code – as in the Hippocratic Oath, if you are a physician – or other potential obligations attached to roles you play.

My point is that morality requires that we look at the broader context in which we act and in which moral decision-making takes place. Moral permissions and authorizations are not plastic key cards that automatically gain us access to what we want. Nor can they be loaned out or transferred to others. Treating them as though they were – or, less uncharitably, as though they were entitlements that could be transferred or exchanged like commodities – is what is wrong with the traditional social and political theories alluded to earlier. They try to justify the state or rationalize war, as though the human rights (and by implication their associated permissions) persons are presumed to have entitling them to do certain things are transferrable simpliciter to others or to collectivities like the state. In the types of case at hand – killing another at his or her behest when (let us assume) it is that person's best judgment that life is not worth living – one cannot abstract the proposed act of killing from its contextual ties. For it is those that are the life-blood of morality.

Thus, the two acts of killing – the primary agent's self-killing, with or without assistance, and the secondary agent's killing of the primary agent – may have different moral assessments. Hence the argument fails.

But it might be argued that even if some killing is morally dissimilar from other killing, there is no moral difference between killing and letting die, and that in many of the most relevant cases regarding this issue the primary agent is seeking assistance in suicide (or is consenting to euthanasia) precisely because he is going to die soon anyway and faces a lot of avoidable suffering in the process. So in these cases the choice facing the secondary agent is either to kill the primary agent (under conditions constituting consensual euthanasia) or let the primary agent die a protracted and painful death against his wishes. If there is no moral difference between killing and letting die, it might be argued, and if in this case one must do one or the other, it is permissible to perform the authorized euthanasia.

This, it should be noted, is a very different argument for euthanasia than we have been considering. If it is sound, it is so whether or not suicide or AS are permissible. So it is essentially irrelevant to the question of whether there is a slippery slope in the moral terrain with which we are concerned. Moreover, if killing and letting die were morally indistinguishable, as the objection would have it, that would tend to support one of my central contentions rather than to undermine it. For then one would have no choice but to look at other morally relevant considerations embedded in the broader context in order to make a decision – either that or flip a coin. Beyond that, it is only true in a relatively inconsequential sense that there is no moral difference between killing and letting die.

Considered abstractively, that is, independently of beliefs, practices, customs, laws, responsibilities and obligations, and even of motives and intentions, there is no difference. But in that sense, there is no moral difference between any two acts. Abstract acts from their context, and describe them in microscopic detail – as but movements of bodies, or more microscopically still, of molecules and atoms, and they are stripped of everything that could give them moral significance. The same with their consequences. Take them, however, in the living contexts in which we encounter them, and they come laden with moral significance. The issue over killing and letting die admits of this solution: considered abstractively, there is and can be no moral distinction between the two. Considered contextually, there is sometimes a moral distinction between them and sometimes not; and when there is, sometimes one is right, the other wrong, and sometimes the reverse. There is nothing more to it than that.

It does not follow from the preceding that euthanasia cannot be morally justified; nothing I have said answers that question one way or the other. All that follows is that it cannot be shown to be permissible by any simple reasoning from the assumed permissibility of suicide, or even of assisted suicide, alone. By extension of the reasoning in connection with Argument C, though I did not detail that extension, it follows more specifically that euthanasia cannot be justified by any simple reasoning from the assumed permissibility of physician-assisted suicide alone. That suffices to show that there is no slippery slope here. If correct, this means that, to make their case, supporters of euthanasia have to do more than just argue for the permissibility of suicide or assisted suicide; and opponents of euthanasia, to make their case, must do more than just argue for the impermissibility of those practices.

University of Rochester
Rochester, New York

NOTES

[1] Physician-assisted suicide is the focus of current debate. But there is no reason why physicians alone should be considered the sole candidates to assist in suicide, if that practice should be justifiable.

[2] In speaking of euthanasia, I am speaking throughout of consensual euthanasia.

[3] In valid arguments it is impossible for the premises to be true and the conclusion false. A valid argument is sound when its premises are true.

[4] This isn't quite true. It does indirectly raise at least one important issue. Some forms of consequentialist reasoning in ethics might have it that, were EU to follow upon the acceptance of suicide and AS, then it would be among their consequences for purposes of moral assessment. This would raise the question, which is of central importance, of what should be counted among the consequences of an action or practice. But as this is a far more complex issue than can be taken up here, I shall not deal with it.

[5] Premise (1) is not meant to imply that suicide is *absolutely* permissible, that is, permissible under all conceivable circumstances. Few but terrorists, for example, would think it permissible to strap explosives to your body and detonate them in a crowded marketplace. Some might object that so-called terrorist "suicide bombings" are not really suicides at all, since the intention is not to kill oneself but to advance a religious and/or political objective, and that it is merely foreseeable that by so doing one will die. To evaluate this contention fully would require a digression into the intricacies of double-effect thinking; I shall assume, with, I believe, support from ordinary language, that such acts qualify as suicides. Those who believe that suicide is permissible typically (though not invariably) think that there is some set of conditions under which killing yourself is permissible—such as that continued life would bring only unrelieved suffering—not that you are justified in ending your own life for any reason whatever.

[7] Suppose that at considerable risk and sacrifice to yourself you save my life on a particular occasion. That arguably creates in me a debt of gratitude to you. Now suppose that one day as I sit by poolside in a recliner reading my newspaper you cry out for help in the center of the pool, and rather than interrupt my reading I ask someone else to toss you the lifeline. Even if that suffices to save your life, I have hardly discharged my debt of gratitude to you – or even acted in a morally decent way. There are some obligations we personally need to carry out and whose discharge we cannot transfer to someone else.

[8] I owe this suggestion to Scott DeVito.

REFERENCES

Nozick, Robert: 1974, *Anarchy, State, and Utopia*, Basic Books, New York.
Walzer, Michael: 1977, *Just and Unjust Wars*, Basic Books, New York.
Washington v. Glucksberg and *Vacco V. Quill*, 521 US—117 S Ct, (1997).

LORETTA M. KOPELMAN

DOES PHYSICIAN-ASSISTED SUICIDE PROMOTE LIBERTY AND COMPASSION?

Discussions about the permissibility of suicide, assisted suicide and euthanasia raise fundamental questions about people's rights, duties, and the meaning of life. Although the issues raised in this debate have been remarkably consistent over the centuries, the contemporary debate seems unique in that many defenders assume that physicians must play a central role in authorizing these procedures. This is evident in the very title of the current debate: should *physician*-assisted suicide be permitted. Yet the justification for physician-assisted suicide can be examined separately from that of assisted suicide, and I restrict my concern to examining two frequently used arguments that physicians and only physicians should have the authority to assist suicide. These arguments are that physician-assisted suicide will first, promote people's liberty and second, foster compassion. I argue that these arguments fail on empirical grounds and because more effective and less contentious means could achieve the same ends.

My objections are not intended to show that suicide or assisted suicide by physicians is wrong *in principle* (or never justifiable under any circumstances). In the past, major figures in philosophy and theology argued that these activities were never justifiable or wrong in principle. Plato, John Locke and Immanuel Kant argued suicide and assisting a suicide were always wrong because they were destruction of God's property. Kant also argued suicide was a degradation of humanity. Aristotle and Thomas Aquinas argued that suicide or assisting in a suicide was a crime against the state.[1] Paul Edward (1998) offers a good review of these and other principled arguments against suicide and assistance of suicide, and of the criticisms that have diminished their influence. In what follows, I do not defend or discuss principled objections to suicide or physician-assisted suicide. Rather, I consider the soundness of two popular arguments that physician-assisted suicide will enhance liberty and promote compassion. I begin with some background information and clarification of terms.

Loretta M. Kopelman and Kenneth A. De Ville (eds.), Physician-Assisted Suicide, 87–102.

1. BACKGROUND: SEPARATING ASSISTED SUICIDE AND PHYSICIAN-ASSISTED SUICIDE

In other times assisted suicide was culturally acceptable and untied to physician's participation. Epictetus (c 55–135AD), a Stoic philosopher and teacher, wrote:

> Upon learning a friend planned to starve himself to death, he went to him on his third day of fasting asking him what had happened to make him choose suicide: "I have decided," he said. "Alright, but what made you decide? For if your decision was the right one, we are at your side and ready to help you make your exit from life." [II.15.7.][2]

Epictetus, was not enthusiastic about suicide, likening it to a soldier abandoning his post.[3] But like other Stoics, he believed that suicide might be a rational option when faced with some dishonor or humiliation worse than death. He praised the athlete who, given the choice of death or castration, chose death as more honorable. Suicide is also a rational option, Epictetus wrote, when one is weary of life's games: "Do not become a greater coward than the children, but just as they say 'I won't play any longer,' when a thing does not please them, so you also, when things seem to you to have reached that stage merely say, 'I won't play any longer,' and take your departure; but if you stay stop lamenting" [I.XXIV.17]. It was part of Epictetus' view of the world that to value finite and perishing things is irrational and we ought to value only those things recommended by reason. When a life cannot be lived with honor, or is no longer worth living, then it is rational to end it, according to Epictetus.

The Stoic view on suicide is not entirely lost. In some cases suicide seems rational and even heroic.[4] Even today we honor soldiers, firefighters or police who sacrifice their lives to save others; we also regard as heroic people who refuse to leave family members to save themselves, thereby facing almost certain death. Such acts are regarded as not only morally responsible but also examples of extraordinary heroism and virtue. The philosopher Immanuel Kant (1775/1980), however, did not regard such heroic and virtuous acts as suicides because he maintained suicides must be ignoble. Yet making acts of suicide wrong by definition ignores arguments that have persuaded many people since ancient times that suicide and assisted suicide can sometimes be justifiable. Consequently, a more neutral definition is offered: Suicide is understood as the voluntary and intentional taking of one's own life (Edwards, 1998). People who cannot tolerate their lives may commit suicide by taking an overdose of their prescribed medicines, slitting their wrists, ingesting poisons, crashing their cars, or leaping from bridges. But according to this definition, police, firemen and soldiers who heroically sacrifice themselves also commit suicide, albeit for very different reasons.

An *assisted suicide* occurs when someone helps another person, by act or omission, to end his or her life voluntarily and intentionally. The individual who assists in a suicide does not kill the person directly but helps the person kill himself/herself. Assistance can take various forms including removing some obstacle, providing the means, or refraining from doing something. *Physician-assisted suicide* occurs when a physician gives assistance to enable someone to bring about his/her own death.

To count as a suicide, assisted or not, the person must be the agent of his/her own death, voluntarily and intentionally. In the clear cases of assisted suicide, persons clearly and unambiguously convey their intentions. Yet many physicians say forthright declarations of intention are often absent and tacit and nonverbal understandings are operative where it is illegal for doctors to assist patients' suicides. For example, to a desperately ill and suffering patient who asks, "How many of these pain killers would do me in," a doctor may say, "Do not take twenty as that would kill anyone." The doctor believes, but does not discuss, that the patient has been collecting the painkillers and is seeking information because she does not want to botch the job. If this is an assisted suicide, then many more physicians have assisted in a suicide than if it is not.

Many of the best known cases of physician-assisted suicide by those favoring such assistance in dying portray physicians as wise, compassionate, and understanding counselors, helping their long-term patients who are suffering terribly and have carefully considered their decisions.[5] Those opposed to physician-assisted suicide tell very different stories such as about ignoble clinicians, or about patients who request assistance when they have been misdiagnosed, lack a home or family support, or mistakenly believe that their suffering is intractable. While these stories favoring or opposing policy permitting assisted suicide may be true and persuasive, the salient question is whether the stories are representative. Because there is as much danger in basing policy on cases as basing scientific generalizations upon them, I try to focus upon aggregate data.

2. LIBERTY ARGUMENTS

A. Defenses of Physician-Assisted Suicide

Many people and societies have well-established moral and social ideals that competent and informed persons have rights to plan and control their lives as long as they do not harm others. Maximizing options for people defends their distinct perspectives and interests, and protects them from social manipulation. One of the most powerful arguments for assisted suicide builds upon these ideals or rights, basing the justification for assisted suicide upon helping people to be in command of their own destiny (Battin, 1982; Brock, 2001; Dworkin et al., 1997). Allowing people the sort of assistance in dying that they choose acknowledges that this is a personal matter that they should control; consequently, the argument continues, we should respect people's choices and allow them to exercise their autonomy by permitting important options, including assistance in suicide. Some rational people wish to avoid suffering physical pain; some find physical and mental deterioration and its disability fates worse than death. Competent, rational, and informed individuals may decide that their lives are no longer worth living and want to plan the time and circumstance of their death.

Acknowledging a right to assistance in suicide, defenders contend, should not affect others because no one would be forced to take such a path or to assist others.[6] Because the liberty of others should be respected as well, none should be required to assist them or participate if they do not wish to do so. It is rational to permit people to decide to end their own lives, defenders argue, when their lives are intolerable, when the person can avoid suffering or what is to them a humiliating existence, and when no one else is affected. That is, if there is a liberty right to assisted suicide, it would be a negative right, or a right not to be interfered with.

How does the argument from self-determination support physician-assisted suicide? A policy legalizing assisted suicide would have to depend upon some institution or profession to administer it. Policy-makers in Holland and Oregon have selected physicians to run their programs. Some see this assistance in suicide as a natural and minor extension of doctors' duties to use the best medical procedures to relieve suffering or promote patient autonomy (Rasmussen, 2000). Presumably when people are contemplating suicide (or refusal of life-saving or important medical care), some knowledgeable professional should evaluate the quality of their decision making. Physicians seem well suited to determine if the person is making an informed, competent, voluntary, and rational decision. Suppose that a person is hospitalized and in such bad shape they may need someone's assistance to find effective means to assist his or her suicide. If physician-assisted suicide were legal, the person's physician could be ideally situated to assist because of familiarity with the person's case, and duties to relieve suffering and be in charge of the case. People thinking of suicide may mistakenly believe that they have an incurable condition or that their pain is intractable; their decisions may be a product of depression, fear or lack of social support.

Advocates of physician-assisted suicide generally favor an array of safeguards including that the person must be terminally ill and competent and that more than one physician confirms the prognosis and approves the request. Physicians can determine if the person thinking of suicide really does so because of a lack of social support, and deal with that problem. If a person is depressed or incompetent, then, according to many defenders of physician-assisted suicide, physicians have a duty to hospitalize them rather than assist them in committing a suicide.

B. Criticisms of Liberty-Right Justifications of Physician-Assisted Suicide

One problem is that many physicians disapprove of assisted suicide, so requiring physician approval could be a substantial obstacle to self-determination. Studies show doctors and nurses overwhelmingly disapprove of or will not participate in activities in assisting patients' suicide (Daly et al., 2000). While this might change if it were made legal, the views of many seem entrenched. Arguably, relying on a physician who objected to physician-assisted suicide would thwart rather than enhance the person's self-determination.

A related problem for this argument concerns aggregate data about the doctor's record in following patients' directives and expressed end of life choices (Teno et al., 1997). If they do not follow patients' wishes very reliably, it seems odd to say self-determination is a key argument for *physician*-assisted suicide. Teno and her colleagues (1997) found that clinicians generally ignored patients' wishes at the end of life: "advanced directives placed in the medical record of seriously ill patients often did not guide medical decision-making beyond naming a health care proxy or documenting general preferences in a standard living will format. Even when specific instructions were present, care was potentially inconsistent in half of the cases" (p. 508). Rather than promoting autonomy, many physicians make assumptions about how patients should want to be treated. Joanne Lynn and her colleagues found despite law or policy on informed consent or advance directives that patients in three countries that were compared, were likely to get standard medical care. "The customization of care to individual patients will be uncommon in all three" (Lynn et al., 1999, p. 282). In short, the large percentage of doctors who ignore patients' preferences or disapprove of physician-assisted suicide probably cannot be counted upon to help patients exercise such a right.

In addition, there is another problem about what it means to have a liberty right. If there is a liberty right to assisted suicide, then the elaborate "protections" often associated with those favoring physician-assisted suicide may appear paternalistic. It seems reasonable to argue that given the finality and irreversibility of the decision someone should check to see if the person is competent, well informed and acting voluntarily. However, some may view these policies as paternalistic. Yet some of the "protections" are unrelated to the quality of the decision. For example, policies often require that the person must be terminally ill. Yet people may also seek assisted suicide not only to avoid the last stages of terminal illnesses, but also to escape mental and physical deterioration from long term, chronic and progressive diseases. If people should be able to plan and control their lives and death, and if death can be a rational escape from dishonorable or humiliating existences, as Epictetus said, why are not the claims of people with degenerative diseases sometimes also compelling? People in early stages of these diseases sometimes foresee a humiliating end to their lives and request assistance in dying when they reach a certain stage of anticipated deterioration, fearing the indignities and dependency associated with dementia from diseases such as Huntington's disease and Alzheimer's disease.[7]

Adults are presumed competent to exercise their liberty rights and the burden of proof is upon others to show they are not. In contrast, suppose that there was a policy that required pre-screening to establish if adults are competent, adequately informed, and making voluntary decisions to vote, marry, or exercise other liberty rights. Whoever did the screening could then easily control people by his verdicts. The analogy, of course, is that physician-assisted suicide gives control to doctors to pre-screen people to exercise so-called liberty rights.

C. Are There More Effective, Less Disruptive Ways to Enhance Liberty?

In selecting a social policy to achieve a certain end, in this case assistance in dying, there is a well-established principle that more effective and less disruptive means are preferable to those that are less effective or more disruptive. Thus, if there are equally effective means to achieve the same end (to aid those seeking assistance in dying) but they are less disruptive or contentious than physician-assisted suicide, then less disruptive remedies are preferable. Gert, Culver, and Clouser (1998) have recently argued that a more effective and less disruptive means exists than physician-assisted suicide to honor self-determination.

A well-established legal and social policy exists that people have a duty to honor people's refusal of medical interventions, and the moral literature also supports their liberty right to refuse medical interventions.[8] In some but not all jurisdictions they can also refuse hydration and nutrition. Gert, Culver, and Clouser (1998) argue that permitting people to refuse hydration and nutrition as well as medication would be a good general policy and undercut the need for physician-assisted suicide. Once refusals or requests are found to be valid, we should honor people's valid refusals of medications, food and water. A chief obstacle to adopting this policy, they argue, is the misconception that death by dehydration or starvation is painful. They argue this is untrue, and the policy should be adopted.

Some may also object to this policy on the grounds that the provision of food and water, even in these extreme cases, has great symbolic importance about compassionate care for people. Yet it would be unjustifiably paternalistic if others' views of what is compassionate defeated someone's informed, competent, and voluntary exercise of their liberty rights. Moreover, a policy of respecting people's valid refusals of hydration, nutrition or medical interventions, I will argue, would be a more effective and less disruptive policy than a policy permitting physician-assisted suicide.

a. More effective. This would be a more effective policy than permitting physician-assisted suicide in that, first, it would probably be more efficient. It is likely that death from dehydration would occur within two weeks, but it might be longer to negotiate and fulfill the various legal and institutional safeguards and reviews favored by advocates of physician-assisted suicide.

Second, it might be more effective in promoting liberty. The policy enhances people's options by its very gradualism. In contrast to interventions that are irreversible and work quickly, withdrawal of nutrition and hydration allows people to reflect and reconsider their choice as the process is set in motion. In addition, it promotes self-determination for all patients and not just those who are terminally ill, as is often the case with policies written favoring physician-assisted suicide. People who are not terminally ill but suffer from degenerative diseases also have rights to refuse these treatments.

b. Less contentious. This proposal to honor people's liberty rights not only seems more effective but less contentious and disruptive. We know many people strongly object to physician-assisted suicide (Daly et al., 2000), yet it is generally agreed that competent, and informed people have the right to refuse medical and other interventions (Gert et al., 1998; Kopelman and DeVille, 2001). This right to refuse medication has been well tested in the courts and reflected in various professional, institutional, and public policies.

Building upon such a policy is less contentious because it would avoid a tangle of arguments about whether or not physician-assisted suicide deeply affects others in the community or advances the interests of the individual ahead of the needs of the community. Even if we establish that someone has a genuine interest for assistance in suicide (or active euthanasia), this does not settle whether their preferences should be honored or if it is a prudent social policy to offer these options.[9] Defenders of physician-assisted suicide, as we have seen, argue that it would not affect the rights or welfare of others. They deny it promotes the view that people ought to be able to get what they want, despite social costs or the impact on professional organizations. But others argue that it undermines key social and professional values, and could affect resource allocation. For example, social policies permitting physician-assisted suicide should require careful review by clinicians since the intervention would be swift and irreversible. Some recommend several physicians or other clinicians review the basis for these decisions. Yet such reviews are costly and some may believe that other demands have greater priority. So even if physician-assisted suicide is justifiable, we can still question if this use of resources is justifiable. Many children (11 million in the U.S. alone) are uninsured and children's most common health problems are easily and inexpensively treated; they include dental pathology, vision impairment, pneumonia, meningitis, allergies, asthma, and hearing loss

(Kopelman and Palumbo, 1997). Parents of these children might prefer seeing resources placed into preventive and treatment programs rather that adding this end-of-life option.

Defenders of physician-assisted suicide, however, might argue these activities are budget neutral or that it might even be cost effective for a society to have physician-assisted suicide. Yet this response would raise another set of concerns about whether assistance in suicide might be encouraged to save money rather than to answer people's needs. Some minority groups already fear the health-care industry for not embracing their best interests. And an alarming number of studies show many biases exist in the way life-saving and costly therapies are allocated to patients (Kopelman et al., 1998). (It is interesting to note that The Netherlands and Oregon have a small minority population.)[10] Physician-assisted suicide programs could undermine community solidarity by funding a controversial program which benefits relatively few when many people have unmet needs.

Thus, the proposal to honor people's valid refusals of nutrition and hydration seems both a less contentious and more effective means of exercising people's autonomy than physician-assisted suicide. It seems more effective in allowing people to consider and carry out their considered judgments. Moreover, if a policy allowing people to refuse medication, hydration and nutrition were fully recognized, a difficult set of considerations could be avoided about whether a physician-assisted suicide policy is socially destabilizing or excessively individualistic or self-interested given social resources. The new laws in Oregon and policies in The Netherlands may help us assess these and other practical concerns about how to evaluate these nonprincipled concerns about physician-assisted suicide (or assisted suicide or voluntary active euthanasia). In the meantime, we can explore what appears to be more effective and less disruptive ways to assist people who wish to end their lives.

To summarize, the liberty arguments for physician-assisted suicide are problematic because they depend upon gaining cooperation from doctors who have a poor record of following people's directives. Moreover, the policies with their build-in safeguards permitting physician-assisted suicide to prevent imprudent, ill-considered, incompetent or nonautonomous requests may seem paternalistic. Finally, a more effective and less disruptive means seems to exist to respect people's liberties in the form of honoring patients' valid refusals of medication, nutrition, and hydration.

3. COMPASSION AND DUTY TO RELIEVE SUFFERING

A. Defenses of Physician-Assisted Suicide

Another influential argument for permitting assisted suicide appeals to people's well-established duties to relieve suffering and treat others with compassion. Assuming that it is sometimes kinder to help a person to commit suicide than to force them to wait until an unavoidably painful disease takes their lives, what evidence is there that physicians should be singled out to assist suicides? One reason is that doctors have ancient and explicit duties to relieve suffering. Established norms of medicine include duties to relieve suffering which in some cases, may be higher than the duty to prolong life. If it is sometimes acceptable to relieve pain and suffering and hasten death by withholding and withdrawing treatments or giving pain medication, then, on this view, active means should also be permitted.

B. Criticisms: More Effective, Less Contentious Means Exist

Once again there appears to be more effective and less contentious social policy to achieve the same ends in the form of either promoting better pain control for people and or honoring their competent, informed and free choices to refuse medical interventions, hydration, and nutrition. Many, though not all patients seeking physician-assisted suicide change their minds when they get good palliative care and pain control (Ganzini et al., 2000), yet studies show clinicians fail to use effective means to fight pain (Resnik, 2001). The Committee on Quality Assurance of the American Pain Society reports "Undertreatment of acute pain and chronic cancer pain persists despite decades of efforts to provide clinicians with information about analgesics" (1994, p. 192). Some estimate that, "pain can be relieved effectively in 90 percent of patients but is not relieved effectively in 80 percent of patients" (Walco et al., 1994, p. 541.) There is already substantial agreement that we need to give clinicians a better education about pain management (American Pain Society, 1994; Field and Cassel, 1997). Recently the Joint Commission on Accreditation of

Healthcare Organizations (JCAHO) unveiled its standards for pain management and identified several barriers to better pain control. These barriers include too little time spent educating clinicians about good pain management, poor clinical training about responding to people's pain, giving pain control too low a priority, and poor skills coupled with limited understanding. President of JCAHO, Dennis S. O'Leary, stated, "Pain control has become a problem because of confusion as to who is responsible [for it], a general lack of knowledge about pain, and misconceptions about drug tolerance and addiction" (Phillips, 2000).

The summary report of the Institute of Medicine's Committee (Field and Cassel, 1997, p. 5) states that the most fundamental deficiency "... in the care of people with life threatening and incurable illnesses [is] too many people suffer needlessly at the end of life, both from errors of omission (when care givers fail to provide palliative and supportive care known to be effective) and from errors of commission (when care givers do what is known to be ineffective and harmful." They agree that the legal, organizational and economic obstacles to providing good pain medications may impede clinicians. Yet "the education and training of physicians and other health care professionals fail to provide them with the attitudes, knowledge, and skills required to care well for dying patients." These are harsh judgments come from extremely prestigious medical and hospital organizations about the skills and attitudes of physicians and other health care professionals about how to relieve pain, provide comfort and palliative care.

There is even a debate among physicians about what means are the most painless and effective way to assist in suicides. Most clinicians use some combination of barbiturates, opioids, and antidepressants (Rasmussen, 2000), but this has proven problematic. Groenewoud and colleagues conclude, "In The Netherlands, physicians who intend to provide assistance with suicide sometimes end up administering lethal medication themselves because of the patient's inability to take medication or because of problems with the completion of physician-assisted suicide" (Groenewoud, 2000, p. 551). Yet some toxins, such as cyanide, are painless, swift, and more effective than routinely used combinations of barbiturates, opioids, or antidepressants. Of course these interventions are more easily obtainable for physicians, but some also explain the reluctance of clinicians to use proven toxins like cyanide. Using barbiturates rather than cyanide preserves the illusion that the primary goal is killing the pain and not the person.[11]

A small group of patients might want physician-assisted suicide even if they were not in pain. Often these are patients who fear losing control over their lives (Sullivan et al., 2000). Some of these people fear future mental or physical pain or deterioration. Yet a more effective and less contentious means also exists for most of these patients in the form of refusal of medication, nutrition and hydration.

A possible objection is that there is no clear line between assisted suicide and giving painkillers or honoring valid refusals of medications, hydration and nutrition. Sometimes forgoing a nourishment or treatments is not so very different from a suicide, and sometimes no clear line can be drawn between giving a pain killer to relieve suffering and giving it to hasten death. Consequently, in some cases it is difficult to draw a bright line between the means having social approval to assist some people in dying (withholding life-saving treatments, letting die, aggressive treatment of pain that hastens death, honoring valid refusals of medication, nutrition and hydration) and those that do not (assisted suicide). Yet the absence of clear lines does not mean things are fundamentally the same. There is no sharp line between blue and green, between green and yellow, between yellow and orange, but there are certainly differences between and blue, green, yellow, and orange. (Some may object that in some cases there is no moral difference in principle between them, but I have conceded this in saying that my objections are not principled.) To summarize, there appear to be less contentious and more effective means to relieve pain and suffering than physician-assisted suicide.

4. CONCLUSION

Empirical evidence from a series of studies raises troubling questions about two frequently used arguments for physician-assisted suicide. The first is based upon promoting people's personal liberty to decide how they want to die. These liberty arguments for physician-assisted suicide are problematic because studies show that doctors have a poor record of following patients' directives and many disapprove of assisting in a suicide. Consequently, seeking their approval or cooperation to exercise what is alleged to be a liberty right, could thwart people's self-determination. Moreover, the policies with their built-in safeguards may seem paternalistic in themselves, or when they impose such requirements that the patient must be terminally ill. Finally, more effective and less disruptive means exist to enhance people's liberties in the form of honoring patients' valid refusals of medications, nutrition and hydration.

A second justification builds upon clinician duties to relieve pain and suffering and holds that physician-assisted suicide is compassionate. Yet, once again, there seem to be more effective and less contentious policy alternatives than physician-assisted suicide. Many, perhaps most, people seeking physician-assisted suicide would want to live if their situation were improved. Yet the data suggests physicians do not do a particularly good job of pain control, and a wide array of options exist to enhance people's situations, including better social support, pain management, and palliative care.

My arguments have focused narrowly on trying to show that liberty arguments and considerations of compassion do not *currently* support physician-assisted suicide. I do not believe assisted suicide is wrong in principle. I do not believe that it is always immoral, unnatural, against God's will, or a sign that the persons seeking it are mentally deranged. I might even agree, moreover, that if anyone should have this authority to assist in someone's suicide, it should be physicians. Given their professional and institutional commitments, they are better suited, for example, than ministers, philosophers or friends to assist them.[12]

Since my opposition does not consist of principled objections, I acknowledge that conditions may change. Future studies might show that doctors carefully follow patients' valid directives, use the most effective pain control measures, and are vigilant in exploring options to relieve suffering. Investigations might also show that physician-assisted suicide is not costly, is necessary to help many patients achieve self-determination and compassionate care, and that other means are less effective, including honoring people's valid refusals of medication, hydration and nutrition. Studies may further show that people are no more fearful of adopting policies permitting physician-assisted suicide programs than withholding or withdrawing of life-saving means, including hydration and nutrition. Under these circumstances a better case might be made for adopting a social policy permitting physicians to assist in people's suicides in order to promote their liberty and treat them with compassion.

Brody School of Medicine at East Carolina University
Greenville, North Carolina

NOTES

[1] Hume's response to these principled arguments was so persuasive that their influence diminished significantly. Like the Stoics, David Hume argued that the act of suicide may be a rational act when life is so cruel, miserable and painful that a person prefers death (Hume, 1777). He argued it does not harm society when the person can no longer contribute to society and their lives are intolerable to themselves.

[2] Epictetus began life as a slave and was so severely abused he lived with severe pain and disability throughout his life. He eventually had a master who recognized his talents, educated and eventually freed him. Epictetus devised many strategies to overcome grief and pain, which are being adapted today in current cognitive therapies to treat depression.

[3] While Kant employs Epictetus' metaphor of suicides being like solders deserting their posts, unlike Epictetus, Kant regards such acts as unjustifiable in all circumstances. Immanuel Kant writes, "We have been placed in this world under certain conditions and for specific purposes. Thus, suicide opposes the purpose of his creator; he arrives in the other world as one who has deserted his post; he must be looked upon as a rebel against God." (Kant, 1774, 1930, 154).

[4] See first century philosophers Seneca and Epictetus.

[5] See, for example, Quill, 1993.

[6] Ikonomidis and Singer, for example, claim liberalism should be understood as, "expressed in terms of negative freedom, rank-order desires, personal identification, and, notably, historical formulation which highlights the broad social embeddedness of the individual." (Ikonomidis and Singer, p. 523).

[7] In addition, still other commentators question why the individual should have to be competent to have this right; if competent people have a right not to suffer, why should incompetent people not have this right as well? Other persons normally can assert liberty-rights on behalf of incompetent persons, and these commentators favor acknowledging that both competent and incompetent people have this right. (Landman, this volume).

[8] See *Vacco v. Quill*, 1997 and *Washington v. Glucksberg* (1997).

[9] For example, many feminists and communitarians reject what they view as the atomistic conception of moral agency inherent in liberalism.

[10] Defendants might respond that people should be no more worried about physician-assisted suicide than about withholding and withdrawing of treatments, which can also be abused or used poorly. Yet there is evidence they fear both, and the latter more than the former. There is growing evidence that physicians may be unjustifiably biased by people's race, age, gender, and socioeconomic background, and that this affects their trust in health care institutions.

[11] Personal communication by Steven Miles.

[12] I am not proposing there should be a policy of minister-assisted suicide, friend-assisted suicide, social worker-assisted suicide, nurse-assisted suicide, or even philosopher-assisted suicide. Nor do I believe that adopting such a policy would lead inevitably down a slippery slope to killing people who were not a nuisance to themselves but to others.

REFERENCES

Angell, M.: 1993, 'Caring for women's health – what is the problem?' *New England Journal of Medicine* 329, 271–272.

The American Pain Society: The Committee on Quality Assurance: 1994, *When Death is Sought: Assisted Suicide and Euthanasia in the Medical Context,* New York State Task Force and on Life and the Law.

Aquinas, T.: 1266–1273, *Summa Theologiae* (IIAIIae.65).

Aristotle: 4th Century, *Nicomachean Ethics* (1138a6-14).

Battin, M.P.: 1982, *Ethical Issues in Suicide,* Engelwood Cliffs, NJ: Prentice Hall.

Brock, D.W.: 2001, 'Physician-assisted suicide – the worry about abuse', this volume, 59–74.

Daly, B.J. et al.: 2000, 'Thoughts of hastening death among hospice patients', *The Journal of Clinical Ethics* 11:1, 56–65.

Dworkin, R. et al.: 1997, 'Assisted suicide: The philosopher's brief', *New York Review of Books* 27 March.

Edwards, P.: 1998, *The Ethics of Suicide,* Routledge Encyclopedia of Philosophy, London and New York.

Epictetus: 1st and 2nd Century, *The Discoveries As Reported by Arrian, The Manual and the Fragments.*

Field, M.J. and Cassel, C.K. (eds): *Institute of Medicine, Committee on Care at the End of Life: 1997, Approaching Death: Improving Care at the End of Life.* National Academy Press, Washington, D.C.

Ganzini, L. et al.: 2000, 'Physicians' experiences with the Oregon Death with Dignity Act', *The New England Journal of Medicine* 342:8 557–563.

Groenewoud, J. et al.: 2000, 'Clinical problems with the performance of euthanasia and physician-assisted suicide in The Netherlands', *New England Journal of Medicine* 342:8, 551–556.

Hume, D.: 1777, *On Suicide,* reprinted in *Hume's Ethical Writings,* edited by Aladair MacIntyre, 1965, Macmillan Company, N.Y., N.Y., pp. 297–306.

Gert, B. et al.: 1998, 'An alternative to physician-assisted suicide: a conceptual and moral analysis', in *Physician Assisted Suicide: Expanding the Debate,* M.P. Battin, Rosamond Rhodes, and Anita Silvers (eds). Routledge, New York and London, 182–202.

The Institute of Medicine: Committee on the Ethical and Legal Issues Relating to the Inclusion of Women and Clinical Trials. *Women and Health Research*: Ethical and Legal Issues of Including Women in Clinical Studies vol.1, eds, AC Mastroianni, R. Faden and D. Federman, Committee on the ethical and Legal Issues Relating to the inclusion of Women in Clinical Studies, Institute of Medicine, National Academy Press, Washington D.C., 1994.

Kant, I.: 1775, 1980, Lectures on Ethics, Translated L. Infield, London.

Komaromy, M. et al.: 1995, 'California physicians' willingness to care for the poor', *Western Journal of Medicine* 162, 127–132.

Kopelman, L.M. et al.: 1998, 'Preventing and managing unwarranted biases against patients', in Laurence B. McCullough, James W. Jones, and Baruch A. Brody (eds.), *Surgical Ethics,* Oxford University Press, Oxford, pp. 242–254.

Kopelman, L.M. et al.: 1997, 'The U.S. health delivery system: inefficient and unfair to children', *American Journal of Law and Medicine* 23, 319–337.

Kopelman, L.M. and Deville, K.A.: 2001 The contemporary debate over physician-assisted suicide, this volume, 1–25.

Landman, W.: 2001, 'A proposal for legalizing assisted suicide and euthanasia in South Africa', this volume, 203–225.

Locke, J.: 1690, Second Treatise on Civil Government, from Two Treatises of Government (§§6, 23, 135).

Lynn, J. et al: 1999, 'Dementia and advance care planning: perspectives from three countries on ethics and epidemiology', The Journal of Medical Ethics 10, 271–285.

Phillips, D.M.: 2000, 'JCAHO pain management standards are unveiled', Journal of the American Medical Association 284: 4, 828–829.

Plato: (4th Century), Phaedo.

Quill, T.E.: 1993 'Barbiturates in the care of the terminally ill', New England Journal of Medicine 328(18): 1350.

Rachel, J.: 1975, 'Active and passive euthanasia', New England Journal of Medicine 292, 78–80.

Rasmussen, P.A.: 2000, 'Physician-assisted suicide and euthanasia', New England Journal of Medicine 343, 150.

Resnik, D.: 2001, 'Physician-assisted suicide: the culture of medicine and the undertreatment of a pain', this volume 127–148.

Seneca: (1st Century) Seneca's Letters to Lucilius.

Sullivan, A.D. et al.: 2000, 'Legalized physician-assisted suicide in Oregon – the second year', The New England Journal of Medicine 342:598–604.

Teno, J. et al.: 1997, 'Do advance directives provide instructions that direct care SUPPORT investigators?', Journal of the American Geriatric Society 45, 508–512.

Timothy, E: 1991, 'Death and dignity: a case of individualized decision making', The New England Journal of Medicine 324, 691–694.

Walco, G.A. et al.: 1994, 'Pain, hurt and harm', The New England Journal of Medicine 331, 541–544.

Vacco v. Quill, 117 S. Ct. 2293 (1997).

Washington v. Glucksberg, 117 S. Ct. 225 8 (1997).

LAURIE ZOLOTH

JOB OPENINGS FOR MORAL PHILOSOPHERS IN
OREGON: PHYSICIAN-ASSISTED SUICIDE AND THE
CULTURE OF ROMANTIC RESCUE

1. INTRODUCTION: KILLING TIME IN GRADUATE SCHOOL:
A MODEST PROPOSAL

As popular discourse considers the issue of suicide in American culture,
we see a range of responses, from the new Hallmark card ("I know that
the Creator has already welcomed your loved one home") to the formal
consideration of the issue by legislatures and courts. Except in Oregon,
the embrace of assisted suicide has not been entirely robust, but as ethicist
Carl Elliott has noted: "while many physicians seem uncomfortable with
the idea ... academic moral philosophers have been prominent in those
who ... seem sympathetic to the idea of physician-assisted death" (Elliott,
1996). Hence, I will consider how to solve the many perplexing problems
raised by the issue and in so doing reflect on the modest question: Why
not philosopher-assisted suicide? In particular, why have only a few
considered the obvious advantages of underemployed moral philosophers
and bioethicists as the best suited to the job of dispatching the patient who
wants not only to die, but to die with the assistance of a well-regarded
(even priestly) professional presence? Oregon, the only state to have
legalized physician-assisted suicide may want to employ them. In
outlining this suggestion, I do not tangentially consider the secondary
benefit of finding a solution to the tightening job market for academically
trained moral philosophers with a specialization in medical ethics.

A. Attributes of the Candidates

Moral philosophers and bioethicists are uniquely suited to reflect on death
and the meaning of life. Unlike, for example, students in engineering or
animal husbandry who spend a great deal of time engaged in the
problems of the concrete and tangible, philosophy and bioethics students
have been drawn to the field despite a veritable thicket of resistance in

Loretta M. Kopelman and Kenneth A. De Ville (eds.), Physician-Assisted Suicide, 103–116.
© 2001 *Kluwer Academic Publishers. Printed in Great Britain.*

our culture to speculative pursuits. Further, moral philosophy, and in particular bioethics, selects for the worried human person. For many in the field, this is not only characterlogical, it has also been a specific and careful aspect of training. Inclinations and natural sympathies, in the Humean sense, also play a key role in the profession; graduate students who are disinclined to worry with sufficient intensity quickly find that they do not do well in our bioethics programs. It is not only the character and inclinations of these worried and sympathetic bioethicists that make them the ideal candidates for their new bedside role, but also the lifestyle that they inhabit. Who else is happy to be drinking coffee and talking endlessly about the meaning of life, the nature of death, and the nuances of suffering in comparative cultural perspectives? Who else will listen to your troubles, and think neither to charge you nor tape you? Moreover, they are possessed of no power that would actually threaten the process of medicine. If a philosopher or bioethicist becomes too troublesome in the hospital or clinic, one can always simply send them back to the academy, where protected by tenure they can construct or decode any theoretical structure without having any effect. Power relationships, whose maintenance is so critical to the functioning of the clinic, are thus maintained.

A further interesting and important feature is the nature of the linguistic encounter itself. While we have seen the fulminating power of the principle of autonomy in many medical contexts, and while we have seen the similar importance to the discourse of futility of the power of beneficence, nowhere but in the physician-assisted suicide discourse has the totalization of the principles themselves been so clear. When one has a liturgy one needs priests, and who better to understand the textual tradition of bioethics than ethicists? Few lay persons use, much less understand, these terms, which accounts for their recitation at every ethics forum – prior to the vulgate discussion.

2. WHY THIS IS NOT SO FUNNY

At this juncture I want to acknowledge that all of the forgoing is meant to be taken as rather a joke, an irony, a mime. I take pains to note this, since just last Sunday The New York Times had a front cover story in the opinion section entitled "Philosophers Ponder a Therapy Gold Mine" (Sharkey, 1998). In that case, it was not a joke, but an account of how philosophers in Germany and New York have begun to "scamper down from the ivory tower and hang out their shingles," a prospect that this author does not find in the least bit amusing. While it is amusing to think anyone would entrust philosophers or bioethicists to assist in suicides, many want to give physicians this authority. My objections to assisted suicide are so fundamental they are not removed by physician special roles or assurances that the person seeking suicide is fully informed, competent, and autonomous. My objections are to the tendency to isolate the act as if it were simply and solely a personal choice.

I want to move in a different direction by beginning with a linguistic costume game: To first ask why it strikes us as funny that philosophers or bioethicists, and not physicians, would do this work, and to claim, as do many sociologists, that what is "funny" displays our deepest cultural tensions, especially our fears about power and uncontrollability. Second, I want to ask with great seriousness what it is exactly that philosophy and bioethics should add to the pointed debates around assisted suicide. Those philosophers and theologians who want to turf this problem to physicians and let them decide when people should have assistance in their suicides have failed in an essential way to make creditable the arguments for justice, for relationality, and for responsible and compassionate actions that ought to be at the foreground of this issue.

The delivery of this paper coincides with the Jewish holiday of Purim, a holiday that on the one hand is a commemoration of the escape from annihilation by the ancient and mythical Jewish community of Shushan, and on the other, a farcical and bizarre carnival in which the celebrants, bedecked in outlandish clothes, are urged to become so drunk that they "cannot tell the difference between Haman (the character of complete evil) and Mordecai, the figure of utter goodness." The masked celebrants, doubly-masked because the traditional outfits are crossed-dressed ones, are urged to perform plays and songs that mock every aspect of the culturally approved decorum, prayfulness, and the rational thought that discerns good and evil. The holiday has a complex relationship to the topic of death. *Purim* is named as such because of the '*pur*,' or lots, that were thrown to decide on the day of the death decree for the Jews. The holiday is exactly one-half year away from the holy-day of Yom Kippur, the solemn day of atonement, fasting, and prayer, in which one also wears a costume of the white *kittel* that traditional Jews wear when they are buried. The rabbinic tradition noted the length between the words (*kippur* and *purim*) and the Purim story is everywhere like the gallows that are built early in the tale, and then wait for use until the final chapter.

A. Death and Control

The effort to legalize physician-assisted suicide is not only about death – it is, like many religious holidays, also about our efforts to control unrelenting tragedy. It is about the meeting of two parallel narratives about what we are and about what we ought to do and be. The first narrative is the increasing surety of the assertion of post-Enlightenment individual rights to possess and control one's own body, narrative, and liberty; it is an argument for individual rights on such issues as abortion, treatment withdrawal, and the empowerment of the patient and the citizens. The demand for the legitimization and the assistance with suicide is another such claim for individual liberty. The second narrative is the increasing linguistic and cultural comfort with the metaphors of medicine and the practitioners of medical science as the expert interpreters and interlocutors for all social problems – even for intimate relationships. At this nexus lies the yearning for scientific, rational, temporal control of the essentially uncontrollable messiness and frailty of being a human person, facing the inevitability of our own death while still working to deny it.

B. Philosophers, Bioethicists, and "De-cloaking"

Why is the suggestion amusing that philosophers or bioethicists deliver assistance in the suicides of the terminally and chronically ill? It is sardonic, in part, because it confronts the real drama and the real stakes of the encounter at the bedside. The joke reveals the death, the sorrow at the heart of narrative of medical technique and legal remedies. This is what bioethicists and moral philosophers, especially post-modern ones, can do well: we deconstruct cover stories.

When we ask about physician-assisted suicide, are we doing more than asking whether it is ever licit for one group of persons to deliberately kill others? We already allow for this in two sanctioned situations – war and capital punishment – so we understand that the moral gesture of killing, by itself, may be permissible in certain settings. (Although in both of these areas, we take special steps to exclude physicians from the act of killing, and we reserve the category of those to be killed to persons whom we name as evil.) When the one to be killed is coincident with the killer, as in suicide, we similarly agree that such an act is sometimes socially permitted, or even necessary. For example, there is rich textual evidence in both the Christian martyrdom and the Jewish Kiddush Hashem tradition that give closely reasoned accounts in antiquity and the medieval period that support suicide. Biblical and Talmudic texts give examples of aid de guerre (Saul), fellow-citizen (Masada), parental (texts of the Crusades), or friend (texts of the Black Death) assisted suicide. When we frame the problem as medical, and offer physicians as the solution, what is it that we are constructing or claiming about our culture?

The medicalization of issues is a social choice in a culture that has turned increasingly to the language of medicine (an "epidemic" of teen violence) and the symbols of medicine (white lab coats on widely varying authorities as a semiotics of power and purity) to understand troubling issues. Suicidal assistance has been framed by other societies in very different ways. In some contexts, cultures have militarized the acts, sending men into futile battles (e.g., Gallipoli). Such acts, by both soldiers and civilians, become not only permitted but also valorized in societies dominated by military referents. At other times, in societies in which religious practice is the heroic deed, suicide is spiritualized, as in the case of fasting women documented in the early Christian era. Finally, in some contexts, suicide has nothing to do with illness or healers at all, but with complex arguments internal to a culture about the relationship to the means of production, or justice considerations (in societies where resources are scarce).

C. Legal Theory as the Basis: The Claim for Autonomy

When the Quinlans turned to the courts to rescue their daughter from the entrapment of her medical technology (after appeals by her priest had failed), they precipitated an escalation of a trend in the emerging field that credited a legal solution to some intractable moral debate. While it may have referred to "prognosis committees" in the dicta, the *Quinlan* court relied on the theory and practice of 18th century social contract and liberty language to frame its decision. It is this language that undergirds informed consent and the first major argument for physician-assisted suicide. What we are claiming is that physicians have duties to the patient that occur within the context of the marketplace, a contractually created environment. The patient, figured as a consumer of an exchanged commodity, healthcare, needs to make an individualistic moral choice with as much information as possible, and without occlusion. Howard Brody frames this first argument thus: "Physicians have a moral obligation to respect the autonomous choices of their patients. Some few patients, even when presented with excellent palliative care, will autonomously select physician-assisted suicide as their preferred option. Physicians should honor that request in those cases" (Brody, 1997).

The mistake is trying to see people stripped of their social relationships. Accordingly, the body can be viewed as a piece of property like any other that can be possessed by the rational, self-regulating self, and that self can negotiate whatever he or she can pay for. On this view, an autonomous self ought to be able to negotiate all the services that a physician can provide, up to and including assistance in a medicalized suicide. Since the foreground story is one of rules, individual rights, and autonomous decisions, safeguards are offered through the informed consent process and licensure of the physician. Elaborate rituals of consent, written consent, contract language of three-day waits that mirror commodity contracts (buyer's remorse clauses) are offered.[1]

The legal gaze operates in another way. When the courts discuss the terminally ill patient, they "see" her like one might "see" a prisoner unjustly held. The linguistic terms stress the horror of death, or the portraiture of a person in solitary confinement, and hence the solutions are extensions of what we allow in the legal system: death can be legal if that is socially required, and wrongs and tragedy can be addressed by recourse to the goods of the marketplace.

This perspective may seem compelling. It is not. Despite over twenty years of debate, the SUPPORT data show that efforts to train physicians to understand the legal injunction to withdraw unwanted intervention have not been successful. It is this ground that locates the debate most fully. Patients report that they are terrified of dying trapped in a painful and humiliated state – hence the very modern demand to die "with dignity" in one's own way and without interference.

The legal gaze is also behind the argument for "decriminalizing" the behavior since "assisted suicide goes on all the time," *sub rosa*, like tax evasion, petty theft, sleeping in parks, or marijuana use. In that construct, if illegal actions are taken for good reasons, the law ought to be changed to make a better fit with the actions, and the assessment of the morality of the behavior is retrospectively altered.

D. The Medical Argument: The Claim for Compassion

Timothy Quill (1991), like Brody, argues that compassionate physicians must be free to act in exceptional cases not only to protect autonomy, but also to fulfill the duties of fidelity. This argument is the second major argument for physician-assisted suicide and rests on another powerful cultural story – that of the intense personal relationship that compels one to break rules, keep powerful, embodied secrets, and become to another "as family" to do the act of great risk against the State, the Church, and previous promises and vows. If we unmask this argument we find a version of the 19th century enthusiasm for romantic, individualistic, love (Rousseauian, Baudelairian).

Prior to the claims of romantic individualism, families were constructed by ongoing communal discourse of transmitted values and obligations. Marriage was nearly universally arranged by elders who loved you, with an attention to a successful union. That same community surrounded the relationship – in birth, illness, and death. But romantic love rests on the early modern notion that aesthetic categories count far more than moral ones, that beauty and desire trump obligation, and that the primacy of the individual over the requirements of the society is clear. Is it any wonder that the increasing isolation of these freely choosing individuals leaves vulnerable persons to face tragedy alone, stripped of the burdens and the benefits of obligatory relationship, with little left but the chance for choice itself?

Many of the texts that promote physician-assisted suicide speak powerfully of the "rare, exceptional case." But, like romantic love, such relationships are rare, capricious, fickle, and essentially personal – one falls in love and devotes a great deal of time to the enterprise, based on attributes of likeness, "attractiveness," or compatibility. Witness the language and hear the stories carefully of Timothy Quill and his Diana whom he assists with her suicide (note the Hellenistically evocative nomenclature). Quill has made us identify with her affliction and made her desire for death recognizable and perhaps even attractive.

Romantic love is narcissistic. If you don't want to fall in love for real and go on the difficult journey that love actually requires, one might still approximate some of the idealized sensations of love through romantic, unrequited, Victorian love. Romantic love is different. Attention to this phenomenon might give us another insight about why the recipients of assisted suicide are so often female. Rescue of the beloved from danger and pain is a familiar theme in the 19th century, with the powerful, expert, and proficient male snatching the woman from the dangers of the painful embodied world. Much more research needs to be done to explore this issue: how the dying are figured as the native savage, and how the patient, read as feminized and hence gendered as female, may become the analogue for the imperiled lover. But the constructs of individual and exceptional romantic love undergird the premise of beneficence and non-maleficence in these heroic stories. It is the doctor, not the patient, who must come to the rescue if the narrative is to be coherent.

The attribute of the modern is in large part an affection for the present moment. Linked to this is the idea that free selves are born with utter voluntariness, and, as such, construct a present self that is an artifice, a work of art. This construct represents an artistic distance from "vulgar, earthly vile nature." This powerful narrative is also operative in the search for the death that is an "elegant" one. Yet, paradoxically, patients must rely on physicians to produce that death.

The intuition that this gesture is not merely love or compassion is buttressed by the real constraints of the physician-patient relationship and of current health care systems. While we hear convincing evidence of compassion, there is no evidence that compassion is a premise, generalizable to the discipline. Have physicians displayed any particular expertise in relieving either their patients' physical or emotional suffering that might further inspire us to support the claim of expertise? It is in large part their failure to do so that has fueled the debate. There is no assurance of access to compassionate care for the chronically ill, to even basic friendly preventative care (much less entrance into the hermeneutic circle of the family), for the far too many Americans without health care coverage. Even with coverage, for seriously ill persons and for most dying patients, the shortened visits, the two-day hospice stays, the panel of shifting doctors is, given the structure of health care, the norm. In most hospice services in California, one can only be admitted to the largely outpatient services if he or she can supply a 24-hour caregiver on site. For the second generation of hospice for the survivors of partners who have died, there is no such person – they lie outside the reach of hospice care. Managed care often further restricts the way that hospice can offer palliation to the poorest patients. The formulary for Medicaid does not include some of the newer and more effective pain medications. Kopelman and colleagues have documented the disturbing tendency for care to vary significantly based on prominity to the caregivers' identity, and the statistical evidence to challenge the claims of a universalizable, compassionate relationship are strong (Kopelman *et al.*, 1998).[2] We are then moved to ask how to address the needs of the many who are in pain, rather than the few who will use the edifice carefully gerry-rigged. The ground shifts under the footing – another California image – the average time that is allowed to be spent with a patient in the large managed care organization in California is seven minutes. A different doctor, usually a resident, sees hospitalized patients. The structure of the project does not allow for the paucity of the emerging medical care delivery system. How different this reality is from the romantic image offered by Brody (1997): that the doctor becomes closely involved, in effect a member of the family during the terminal phase of dying. (All of which is hard to do in seven-minute office visits.)

Finally, if the relief of pain is a central concern, then why is the category of persons that might be killed restricted to only the terminally ill within rather narrow guidelines?[3] It is critical to remember the last major public policy debate on euthanasia was fueled not by rights or autonomy at all, but as a result of desperate pleas for compassion for a child, Peter Knuer, born in 1933 with seizures and severe spina bifida.

If assisted suicide is an expression of compassion, why are physicians the only ones with the mandate to provide what would seem to be an essential human duty, especially since relieving suffering, primarily and hitherto, is the function of the family? It is no doubt true, in some restricted physical sense, that suffering is equated with pain as long as doctors hold sole licensure to the best drugs. But suffering is a far broader category, and Brody contends that doctors have some special role in its relief, which is not at all self-evident. Why should the suffering of the ill, beyond the narcotizing of pain receptors, be in the hands of physicians as opposed to others, especially persons in role-specific relationships that attend to suffering, such as parents, spouses, lovers, friends, or one's religious community?

In part, this is linked again to the narrative of romantic love. Once medicine became organized in such a way that the dying were placed more conveniently in hospitals, ICUs, and nursing homes (places where families, much less groups of friends, are often uneasily tolerated), the physician or nurse became the central person, the priest who is "in the house" of the dying. Once societies become convinced that faith is a pleasant, but extraneous enterprise in the sphere of health care, there is no moral point to the witness of death by the person's spiritual community; death becomes un-witnessed, and unfamiliar.

Why do we want physicians to have such roles in the first place? As high priests of the hospital and clinic, they do tend to be around at the time that a person is very sick, of course, but they are hardly the ones who give the backrub, or even administer the drugs. The physician is usually an intermediary in real terms, between the pharmaceutical distribution industry and the nurse. But what the physician can provide, which no one else possibly can, is the order. This reality ought to direct our attention to the real worth of the intervention. If the suicidant is not a secret poison, stored illicitly, but a medication, prescribed in Latin over a coded number, then it is something with great power. This drug, after all, is the same as that which would be hoarded by a patient. But the ordered quality is what is sought, and what is paradoxically comforting. Medicalized, the performative sign is transformed from an outlaw desperate gesture to a sanctioned alternative, one that can be chosen and then purchased at the drug store as a customer. In a search for expertise, the talisman of trust is experience. Brody (1997) offers the doctor as the one who will not panic or be stopped by death, and who asks, "wait a minute . . . what are we doing here? Ought I to be doing this?"

The most forceful arguments in favor of physician-assisted suicide, such as that offered by Quill, portray an ideal of compassionate, committed, and knowledgeable doctors (pictured as vertical and gendered as male) providing help and counsel to desperately ill patients (pictured as horizontal, gendered as female). But there is barely time to reflect carefully on the issue. If there were, the argument for compassion would have a different ending. After the death is ordered, the doctor would not hurry to the next patient but would help hold the family together. When we speak of solidarity and friendship, we need to wonder aloud about who would come after the medication is delivered. Who sits by the bedside, who cleans the sweat-soaked sheets? The nurse, of course, and the family. After the death it is the family and spiritual community who are left to pick up the cadaver and piece their lives together.

We find the problem of physicians-as-assistors especially problematic when we look at the history of the dying patient. Physicians, classically seeing death as a looming defeat created a "team" to "fight" death. When death seems to be "winning" the denouement is troubling. Patients are too often made into a battleground.

This mythology squares with the insistence that only physicians would possibly have the expertise to administer the *coup de grace* skillfully enough; yet we do not find data that supports that contention either. Physicians sometimes seem to shy away from the most efficient and painless means of assisting death in favor of less effective means, typically drugs to assist sleep. Many commentators have noted that cyanide is swift and painless, yet often rejected in favor of barbiturates, which are less certain in their reactions. Are they preferable only because they are routinely used medicine, and thus more easily obtained? Kopelman suggests not. "Using barbiturates rather than cyanide preserves the illusion that the primary goal is killing the pain and not the person (Kopelman, 2001)." This might explain why clinicians may prefer something that appears to be a standard medication rather than a proven toxin. Standard protocols for animals include concentrated doses of barbiturates combined with toxins. Knowledge of fatal dosages is readily available to physicians, and even to some philosophers, and despite Brody's argument, such doses require no special expertise to administer. Caregivers have been taught, since the advent of managed care, to deal with far more complex medical maneuvers than this.

E. For What Can We Hope?: The Claim of Moral Philosophy

I want to turn again to a larger framing comment – the necessity of humility for everyone, physicians, nurses, lawyers, philosophers and bioethicists in the face of this debate. Two days prior to the delivery of this paper, I witnessed a horrific car crash, got out of my car, ran to the scene, and said "I am a nurse, can I help?" Now, I did not say, "I am a Moral Philosopher," or "I am a Philosopher." Instead, I felt for pulses, started CPR, on my knees, in the street. The woman lay dying before us, blue, staring, the purse of her body filling with blood. We did OK, I found the thick beat of her heart again under my hands. But I thought of how rare it is that moral philosophers see the blue face of death. I raise this cautiously not to heroicize it, but for the opposite reason – it made me ashamed to be writing a jokey, clever, remote paper – it overwhelmed me. It is that reality that Carl Elliott asks us to remember in his ironic piece on philosopher-assisted suicide when he argues: get that academic who thinks this assistance is a good idea to carry the load. "If (it) is genuinely praiseworthy from an ethical point of view, carrying it out should reflect well on philosophy" (Elliott, 1996). It is a humility that one could hear more of.

Justice and compassion can be dwarfed by romantic notions of rescue. Romantic rescue is not a bad thing, but, like passionate hate, it is not the best way to construct social and medical practices. Patients are usually strangers to clinicians. Doctors' encounters with these vulnerable strangers should exist within the narrative frame of justice. And the reality that underlies even the nicest physicians' interventions is that after the death, unlike the real family, the physician will be paid, and then move along to the next patient.

F. Struck by the Lightning of Possible Storms: The Argument from Moral Philosophy

Foucault, in an essay called "the masked philosopher," offers the following definition of the task of philosophy:

> I was saying just now that philosophy was a way of reflecting on our relationship to truth. It should also be added that it is a way of interrogating ourselves: if this is the relationship that we have with truth, how must we behave?

This embrace of the darker world of disconcerting instability, the "lightening of possible storms" (Foucault's term) is an embrace of the tragedy of the individual and of the way that particularity resists, finally, our attempts to normalize it – death resists the clinical gaze, if we allow it to strike us, clean through. In this view, we should allow death to be overwhelming, to stun us, and to be in the hands of the families and friends who will not only clean up after, but live, not in the continuous present, but in the life after death that the physician will leave.

Bioethicists or philosophers, could, of course, as Elliott reminds us, do the trick as surely as physicians. They might even make better friends. But it is my contention not simply that we should reject that role entirely for doctors, philosopohers, bioethicists or others. Rather, we should reject assisted suicide as a justifiable option and see we have serious work to do at the figurative bedside, the hard work of social ethics and justice theory. For if we are to be attentive to trouble the discourse of the particular, remain sensitive to the fact that the structure erected in the name of the marketplace and romantic love is desperately unstable, what else can we do? We know what lawyers do – they turn to the legal contract or the lawsuit.

Foucault suggests another direction – to turn from the aesthetic categories of modernity itself. This will mean a direct encounter with the instability of the shifting ground, a recognition that, in his words, "the world is in error." We must also call attention first to the deep injustice of the terrain of health care prior to building the edifices for a few. Philosophy can offer compelling attention to the problems inherent in how the arguments are made, as well as identifying whose interest and telos they might co-incidentally serve. We can offer a close textual attention to the foundational narratives that argue for this fundamental change in the performative gesture of medicine itself, and we can parse their embedded meanings and implications.

But ultimately we fail if we do not raise determined philosophic queries about why there is such demand for this service at a point in American social history when justice in access to essential health care services is wanting, and when illness itself is so closely associated with race, class, gender, and marginalized status. We must recognize that we cannot agree that even seemingly reversible and benign interventions, such as birth control and prenatal incentives, are free of racial biases. In terms of our California metaphor, what starts out as careful construction ends up as trailer parks for the poor, done cheaply, done just well enough. We might ask for attention to the persistence of discrimination toward the disabled, and the studies that remind us that all health care providers are poor judges of the life experience of the disabled, before we embark on construction of a whole hillside of houses in a place we can predict will be at risk.

The hard pursuit of justice ought to strike us like lightning – illuminating the terrain with clarity. Romantic love is about the needs of each, but social justice is about the needs of all. Love can be unrequited, you barely need another. But justice requires a community. You must have a discourse and competing moral claims. Attention to the possible and not only the present, but the past and the future as well, saying "wait a minute, what are we doing here?" is not only the question of the family, it is our question as philosophers, as well.

San Francisco State University
Berkeley, California

NOTES

[1]   Another correlate of the way that we see the emergence of the totally autonomous citizen stripped of family and community is in the growing numbers of homeless.

[2]   In fact, Kopelman *et al.* (1998) draw our attention to the very way that doctors misread and mistreat the health care needs of those who are disempowered. Rather than promoting autonomy, many physicians make assumptions about how patients want to be treated. She writes, "there is growing evidence a physician may be unjustifiably biased by people's race, age, gender, socioeconomic background in directing patients' care and treatments." Gornick and her associates analyzed the 1993 Medicare data, the most recent available, comparing it to 1990 census data to compare the health care of 24.2 million whites and 2.1 million African-Americans. Despite similar insurance coverage they found that income, race and gender affect how patients receive costly, scarce, or life-saving resources. African-Americans were 33% less likely to undergo cardiac catheterizations, 44% less likely to undergo angioplasty, and 54% less likely to undergo coronary artery bypass graft (CABG). They were also more likely to have procedures most people would prefer to avoid, such as hysterectomies and amputation. In an editorial published on this study, Geiger notes the disturbing conclusions that African-Americans with comparable insurance are less likely to receive renal transplants, receive hip or total knee replacements, and undergo gastrointestinal endoscopy, among other procedures, but are more likely to undergo hysterectomy and amputation. She correctly pointed out the "consistency of these findings with a growing body of evidence of unwarranted bias in medicine. Other studies suggest disturbing patterns of unjustified bias by clinicians against those who are female, poor, elderly, Latino, and African-American. Three studies report that equally qualified women are less likely than men to have major procedures for diagnosis or therapy of coronary heart disease or to take part in clinical trials with their important health opportunities." (Kopelman, 2001)

[3]   Kopelman (2001), this volume, agrees that compassionate and knowledgeable physicians often assist in suicides to relieve pain. She argues they might, however, do a much better job of relieving pain.

REFERENCES

Brody, H.: 1997, 'Assisting in patient suicides is an acceptable practice for physicians', in R. Weir (ed.), *Physician-Assisted Suicide*, Indiana University Press, 107–135.

Elliot, C.: 1996, 'Philosopher assisted suicde and euthanasia', *British Medical Journal* 313, 1088–1089.

Kopelman, L.M.: 2001, 'Does physician-assisted suicide promote liberty and compassion', this volume, pp. 87–102.

Kopelman, L.M. *et al.*: 1998, 'Preventing and managing unwarrented biases against patients', in Laurence B. MCCullough, James W. Jones, and Baruch A. Brody (eds), *Surgical Ethics*, Oxford University Press, Oxford, pp. 242–254.

Quill, T.E.: 1991, 'Death and dignity: a case of individualized decision making', *New England Journal of Medicine* 324(10), 691–4.

Sharkey, J.: 1988, 'Philosophers ponder a therapy gold mine', *New York Times*, March 8, 4:1.

PART III

PHYSICIAN-ASSISTED SUICIDE:
VIEWS FROM THE CLINIC

GAIL J. POVAR

PHYSICIAN-ASSISTED SUICIDE:
A CLINICIAN'S PERSPECTIVE

Ten physicians sit around the polished conference table, talking earnestly, each visibly uncomfortable. The subject is physician-assisted suicide; the goal to provide ethical guidance on the subject for a large and influential organization of physicians. On some aspects of the topic, there is consensus. We agree that comfort and palliation should always be provided, and that such care should, for most patients, erase the need to consider suicide. We also agree for the most part that there are convincing moral and ethical arguments against physician-assisted suicide. And yet, there is profound hesitation to state that, as a matter of public policy, physician-assisted suicide should be considered a criminal offense.

It is not a matter of colleagues protecting other colleagues who act wrongly. Rather, there is a profound sense of respect for and humility in the face of others' suffering and the moral obligation of the physician to alleviate suffering as much as possible. And there is awareness that for all our knowledge about palliation, pain is not the only or even the most important issue in many patients' interest in suicide.

And so we struggle. Many of us carry within us a story of a patient or a family member, a story that will not allow us the comfort of uniform condemnation of a practice whose wrong or rightfulness seems to rest so completely on the particulars. The committee is caught within the tension between philosophical arguments about physician-assisted suicide as a matter of policy, and the character of physician-assisted suicide as a phenomenon of private lives and relationships. Physicians must live within this tension whenever a patient asks "can you help me?"

1. PRIVATE RELATIONSHIPS, PUBLIC CONSEQUENCES

It is not difficult to identify the egregious situations that engender wholesale rejection of physician-assisted suicide. The *deus-ex-machina*-like interventions of Kevorkian, for instance, bear no resemblance to clinical medicine provided in the context of a durable and committed, doctor–patient relationship (Quill, 1995). Yet, even in situations where

Loretta M. Kopelman and Kenneth A. De Ville (eds.), Physician-Assisted Suicide, 119–126.
© 2001 *Kluwer Academic Publishers. Printed in Great Britain.*

the relationship apparently exists, as in the Netherlands, some find evidence of a slippery slope from limited application to less cautious and perhaps less patient-initiated assisted euthanasia (Henk and Welie, 1992). Still others have pointed out that, whether or not the data demonstrate abuse, legal affirmation of access to physician-assisted suicide is immoral because it fundamentally contradicts and undermines the role of the physician as healer (Singer, 1990). To most physicians, such arguments convincingly override those advocating permissiveness toward physician-assisted suicide, whether they are based on grounds of autonomy or on comparability to withholding life-sustaining treatment (Brock, 1992). Yet, many of those same physicians are loathe to recommend statutory intrusion into this aspect of doctor–patient decision making.

One explanation for this reluctance is the physician–patient relationship itself. Physicians who distinguish between themselves and Dr. Kevorkian, yet who publicly advocate for permission to engage in physician-assisted suicide, emphasize the centrality of a meaningful physician–patient relationship to any such decision. Indeed, the relationship that is a *sine qua non* of justifiable physician-assisted suicide also may provide the best protection against unwarranted choice of such a path (Quill, 1992). A physician who knows the patient well can identify factors such as depression, cognitive change, or external stresses, including inadequate pain management, which might lead the patient to request assistance in dying, however contrary to his or her own stated values or interests. In such instances, the fact that the physician is not *a priori* opposed to physician-assisted suicide lends credibility to his or her efforts to dissuade a patient from an irrevocable decision at a particular moment of frustration or remediable misery. Appropriate management of pain and disability is the first duty of the physician, no matter what else follows. Yet fear of legal intrusion into the relationship, whether through monitoring of prescribing practices or investigation of means of death, may nevertheless prevent some physicians from treating the patient optimally. The appropriate management of pain blurs into the management of death.

2. MANAGING PAIN, MANAGING DEATH

Barely 70, she lies quietly, day after day. Although cancer cells originating in her breast now eat at bone everywhere, morphine and sedation have smoothed the pain lines around her mouth. But control of the pain has left her silent and unresponsive. Cancer has not invaded her heart, which keeps beating day in and day out, and her hearty, smoke-spared lungs breathe on despite the malignant fluid collection that obliterates much of the room in half her thorax. Day after day, I go in and talk softly with the exhausted family who have sat by her bedside in shifts, not wanting her to die alone. When they ask "Is there anything you can do to make her more comfortable?" we all know the question they are really posing. "No," I answer. "She seems not to be in pain."

Perhaps the most profound effect of the physician-assisted suicide movement has been enormously increased attention to pain management and palliative care. Although the pharmacodynamics of morphine, and appropriate dosing have been well understood for decades, physicians often avoided using appropriate doses of these drugs to relieve pain for fear of being accused of having brought about the death itself (Buchan and Tolle, 1995). The hospice movement, and more recently, the advent of palliative care as a medical subspecialty, have both altered and reflect profoundly changed attitudes over the last two decades toward pain management, particularly in terminally ill patients.

The principle of double effect is perhaps the philosophical precept most frequently invoked to justify the use of large doses of narcotics to assuage pain, even if, in so doing, death is brought closer. But physicians, watching families wait day after day for a loved one's death after much suffering and many tears, are only too aware that the distinction between achieving pain relief and deliberate hastening of death is not so easily drawn. Relief is sought not only from pain, but from the extension of existence. Physicians have heard too many dialysis patients not only request release from the burden of dialysis, but also from the life of a dialysis-dependent person. The language is not merely "please, let me stop dialysis." The words are "please, let me die." Although philosophers may argue that the disease, not the doctor, caused the death, when we disconnect the respirator, it very much *feels* as though we have, at least, issued death an engraved invitation (Povar, 1990). When our action follows the family's request: "please – he would not want to live like this, he always said to let him die," and we offer terminal sedation to protect the patient against the horrors of suffocation, physicians sense that we are also protecting at one time the patient, the family, and ourselves from an unexpected and unwanted survival (Truog *et al.*, 1991). Neither causation nor intention are so easily parsed as to offer medical or philosophical shelter from ambiguity regarding physician-assisted suicide under these circumstances. It seems clear that the physician has not only prevented suffering, but assured a good death.

Other social and economic factors make it harder in the individual circumstance to condemn physician-assisted suicide, despite our knowledge of appropriate care of the dying (Council on Scientific Affairs, 1996). Prognosis of survival in the patient with metastatic cancer is imprecise, until the last 6-8 weeks. Yet hospice benefits are typically only available for six months. Ironically, patients admitted to hospice may survive longer than expected, due to the improved psychological and physical condition associated with better pain management. Yet, few families can afford to pay for hospice out-of-pocket. As a result, physicians and families are faced with a peculiar "survival deadline" imposed by insurance constraints. In other contexts, rural environments for example, hospice care may be difficult to find in any form. Inpatient hospice care may require tearing the patient away from home and loved ones, yet geography, economics, and scarcity of personnel make home hospice care difficult. Although physician-assisted suicide in such contexts in effect enables an inadequate system to persist, the physician is torn between her clinical role as healer, her social role as an agent of change, and compassion for the suffering of the family and patient before her. Would it make sense to compound the inequities of the system by putting a physician who was willing, under such conditions, to participate in physician-assisted suicide at risk for a charge of murder?

3. DEATH AS COMFORTER, DEATH AS COMPLICITOR

A 74-year-old former university professor has watched several aunts and uncles, and his mother die of medical complications of dementia. His vivid memories of frustration, anger, confusion and grief during the course of their illnesses profoundly color his views about his own aging and death. Most of all, he dreads becoming someone else, and having his children's father replaced by a person neither he nor they would recognize. He worries about being a burden, and about using up resources his grandchildren could put, in his view, to better use. In unsparing language, he asks his physician to help him ensure that he will not live to become an alien, burdensome stranger should he develop dementia.

Bearing witness to the suffering of patients with irremediable conditions influences many a clinician. As physician Eric Cassell eloquently observes, "the warrant of medicine in every culture is the universal existence of sickness and suffering and the need for relief" (Cassell, 1991). Not all suffering is treatable with pain medications or sedation, however. Suffering may be brought about by "... the impending threat to the integrity or continued existence of the whole person" (Cassell, 1991, p. 24).

Many physicians share with their patients a dread of decrepitude. Doctoring the frail or demented elderly cannot help but confront the physician with the absence of adequate social support for families, the expense and relative scarcity of truly excellent care for such patients. The experience of seeing one person slowly and unrelentingly replaced by another, often distant, withdrawn and unknowing, is profoundly saddening. We watch families care for someone they do not know, out of respect for the person that used to be. The elderly watch this phenomenon around them with great concern. Is it surprising then, that a patient might wish to take advantage of the fact that "... dementia provides a window of time in which the person still directs his own existence and when it is no longer his own?" (Buchanan, 1989).

For physicians, these cases are in many ways more difficult than those involving terminally ill cancer patients for whom morphine offers respite, or respirator patients whose suffering can be ended by withdrawal of medical intervention. For these latter, we can honestly argue that the disease will follow an inexorable course, that the period of burden need not last long, and that we have the tools to ameliorate suffering. But for patients with chronic, gradually destructive illnesses, such assurances are not so easily given. The suffering in the case of the patient on the verge of progressive dementia is existential, involving complex concerns regarding loss of self, fear of being a burden to others, and even a perceived "duty to die" among those with a commitment to a particular notion of inter-generational justice (Hardwig, 1997).

We appropriately recoil at the idea of assisting someone to die who is still very much a communicative, functional individual, but find ourselves deeply conflicted by the argument that physicians can assure a "good death" in a way that the patient cannot. Avoiding the "prolongation of dying" and "achieving a sense of control" are essential dimensions of end-of-life care in patients' eyes (Singer *et al.*, 1999). Inevitably, some patients' concerns about control over the time and manner of death, especially in the face of actual or anticipated suffering, should lead to conversations with their physicians about physician-assisted suicide. If we do not agree to the request, we risk the possibility that such patients will choose to die at their own hands much earlier than might otherwise be the case.

Philosophers Dan Brock and Allen Buchanan argue that we can override the "dispositive property right" of a person's "surviving interests" over the "living, sensing body" that is no longer that person only to avoid some very important harm (Buchanan and Brock, 1989, p. 166). Indeed, those with dementia and other chronically disabling diseases are precisely the population at greatest risk of abuse through an overly liberal social policy or attitude toward physician-assisted suicide. The slope from respecting a patient's uniquely difficult situation toward a general lessening of concern or care for such patients is clearly very slippery. Moreover, honoring an individual's request for physician-assisted suicide when the prompt is fear of dementia confirms the patient's perception that such a state is unalterably negative and unpleasant, and implies that there are no alternatives to the demeaning existence the patient envisions. Once again, the physician is enabling an unsatisfactory status quo. In the face of these potential harms, the need for a firm policy against physician-assisted suicide seems obvious. But we should acknowledge that such a policy will have unintended consequences for individuals, families, and physicians that are profoundly unsettling. As ever longer life and longer periods of frailty characterize our population, physicians will encounter more and more patients making the same request as the university professor. How shall we answer them?

4. SOLACE

For the individual physician, talking quietly with a patient he has known for a long time, the answer to a request for physician-assisted suicide will never come easily. The moral position may be clear, but the good answer less so. While saying no, we must still, somehow, be able to respond meaningfully to the suffering that begets the request. Public policy must protect the vulnerable, but private acts must offer solace. While the medical tools to care for those in pain are more than adequate, the capacity to respond to the myriad forms of suffering that physicians encounter remains inadequate. The ongoing difficulty of the struggle manifests itself in recent articles suggesting that terminal dehydration may straddle the disputed boundary between death caused by the physician and death caused by the disease (Miller and Meier, 1998). Regulatory barriers to appropriate use of pain medication persist, and lack of access to adequate care remains a legitimate fear for many patients (Tolle, 1998). Finally, we are only beginning to address the psychological and social structures, and the moral language necessary to support physicians, families, and patients coping with dementia in meaningful ways (Journal of Clinical Ethics, 1998). In the meantime, many physicians will find themselves on the one hand publically and sincerely opposing physician-assisted suicide as a matter of policy, while privately shielding from rebuke those colleagues who, having truly done all else they could and faced with tragedy wherever they turn, provide patients with the means to die in peace.

REFERENCES

Brock, D.: 1992, 'Voluntary active euthanasia', Hastings Center Report 22, 10–22.
Buchan, M.L. and Tolle, S.W.: 1995, 'Pain relief for dying persons: dealing with physicians' fears and concerns', Journal of Clinical Ethics 6, 53–60.
Buchanan, A.E and Brock, D.W.: 1989, Deciding for Others: The Ethics of Surrogate Decision-Making, Cambridge University Press, Cambridge.
Cassell, E.: 1991, 'Recognizing suffering', Hastings Center Report 21, 24–31.
Council on Scientific Affairs: 1996, 'Good Care of the Dying Patient', Journal of the American Medical Association 275, 474–477.
Hardwig, J.: 1997, 'Is there a duty to die?', Hastings Center Report 27, 34–42.
Henk A.M.J. and Welie, J.V.M.: 1992, 'Euthanasia: normal medical practice?', Hastings Center Report 22, 34–43.
Hendin, H., Rutenfrans, C., and Zylica, Z.: 1997, 'Physician-assisted suicide and euthanasia in the Netherlands: lessons from the Dutch', Journal of the American Medical Association 277, 1720–1722.
Miller, F. G. and Meier, D.E.: 1998, 'Voluntary death: a comparison of terminal hydration and physician-assisted suicide', Annals of Internal Medicine 128, 559–562.
Pellegrino, E. 'Doctors must not kill', Journal of Clinical Ethics 3, 95–102.
Povar, G.J.: 1990, 'Withdrawing and withholding therapy: putting ethics into practice', Journal of Clinical Ethics 1, 50–56.
Quill, T.E. and Cassel, C.K.: 1995, 'Nonabandonment: a central obligation for physicians', Annals of Internal Medicine 122, 368–374.
Quill, T.E., Cassel, C.K., and Meier, D.: 1992, 'Care of the hopelessly ill: proposed criteria for physician assisted suicide', New England Journal of Medicine 327, 1380–1383.

Quill, T.E., Meier, D.E., Block, S.D., and Billings, J.A.: 1998, 'The debate over physician-assisted suicide: empirical data and convergent views', *Annals of Internal Medicine* 128, 552–558.

Singer, P.A., Martin, D.K., Kelner, M.: 1999, 'Quality end-of-life care: patients' perspectives', *Journal of the American Medical Association* 281, 163–168.

Singer, P. and Siegler, M.: 1990, 'Euthanasia: a critique', *New England Journal of Medicine* 322, 79–81.

Tolle, S.W.: 1998, 'Care of the dying: clinical and financial lessons from the Oregon experience', *Annals of Internal Medicine* 128, 567–568.

Truog, R., Arnold, J.H., and Rockoff, M.A.: 1991, 'Sedation before ventilator withdrawal: medical and ethical considerations', *Journal of Clinical Ethics* 2, 127–128.

1998, *Journal of Clinical Ethics* 9. This entire special issue deals with the broad spectrum of challenges faced in caring for patients with dementia.

DAVID B. RESNIK

PHYSICIAN-ASSISTED SUICIDE: THE CULTURE OF
MEDICINE AND THE UNDERTREATMENT OF PAIN

1. INTRODUCTION

Pain control is one of the key points of contention in current debates
about physician-assisted suicide. Defenders of physician-assisted suicide
argue that a competent patient's desire to relieve intractable pain and
suffering is a compelling reason for permitting this practice (Quill et al.,
1992; Brock, 1993; Quill et al., 1997). Opponents contend that physician-
assisted suicide is not required to relieve pain and suffering because these
symptoms can almost always be controlled with good pain management
and palliative care (Singer and Siegler, 1990; Emanuel, 1998; American
Medical Association (AMA), 1997). Both sides of this issue acknowledge
that it is important to offer patients quality end-of-life care, including
adequate pain control.

Questions about medicine's ability to relieve pain and suffering are
empirical issues that can be settled by more scientific data about the
causes of pain and the analgesic effects of medications and surgery. In the
last two decades, clinical researchers, neurologists, oncologists,
psychologists, and pharmacologists have accumulated a great deal of
evidence about pain assessment and treatment (World Health
Organization, 1990; Agency for Health Policy and Research, 1994).
There also now exists a huge body of literature describing methods for
quality end-of-life and palliative care (AMA, 1997; Harrold and Lynn,
1998; Byock, 1997; Ingham and Foley, 1998; Lynn and Wilkinson,
1998).

In the last few years, many institutions, such as hospices, the Robert
Wood Johnson Foundation, pain initiatives, the American Cancer Society,
the AMA, medical boards, and state legislatures, have stressed the
importance of palliative care in the treatment of the terminally ill in order
to help patients make the transition from life to death without resorting to
physician-assisted suicide (Horgan, 1997; DeShano, 1997; AMA, 1997;
Martino, 1998). Many writers have argued that we should improve

Loretta M. Kopelman and Kenneth A. De Ville (eds.), Physician-Assisted Suicide, 127–148.
© 2001 *Kluwer Academic Publishers. Printed in Great Britain.*

palliative care as a way of decreasing the demand for physician-assisted suicide (Foley, 1997; Emanuel, 1998). The palliative care movement has also had some impact on medical education and research. For example, medical and nursing schools now routinely introduce their students to pain assessment and treatment techniques, many physicians specialize in pain treatment, and a variety of new methods of pain control have been explored in recent years.

This knowledge has not yet had a transforming effect on clinical practice, however, and the fear of inadequate pain control is frequently cited as a key factor in the demand for physician-assisted suicide (Emanuel, 1998). One of the most notable findings of the Study to Understand Prognoses and Preferences for Outcomes and Risks of Treatments (SUPPORT) is that 40% of patients in end-of-life situations report severe pain most of the time (SUPPORT Principal Investigators, 1997). Many patients with terminal (and non-terminal) illnesses find suicide to be a palatable alternative to severe pain, and about two-thirds of oncology patients find physician-assisted suicide acceptable for people with unremitting pain (Sullivan et al., 1997; Goldstein, 1997). In a study of the practice of physician-assisted suicide and euthanasia in the United States, 97.4% of oncologists who admitted to participating in either of these practices reported that their patients were experiencing unremitting pain (Emanuel et al., 1998).

The problem of inadequate pain control goes beyond end-of-life care, however. Some studies show that other types of pain, such as cancer pain (Cleeland et al, 1994; 1998), trauma pain (Todd et al., 1993), post-operative pain (Ng et al., 1996), and chronic pain (McGivney and Crooks, 1984) are also undertreated. Studies also indicate that there are racial, ethnic and gender differences in the adequacy of pain control (Todd et al., 1993; Ng et al., 1996).

While many health care professionals are aware of the importance of pain control in treating terminally ill patients, pain is still routinely underreported, underdiagnosed, undertreated, and underfunded (Horgan, 1997; Goldstein, 1997; Martino, 1998; Jost, 1998). One of the tragedies of end-of-life care is that so many people view physician-assisted suicide as a reasonable alternative to unrelenting pain, even though the empirical evidence shows that a vast majority of terminally ill patients do not have to spend their final days this way (Agency for Health Policy and Research, 1994; Atkinson and Davies, 1993; Byock, 1997; Lynn and Wilkinson, 1998).

The purpose of this paper is to shed some light on the causes of this tragedy by exploring how the culture of modern medicine responds to pain. Since clinicians now have the technical means to control pain in most cases and to provide quality end-of-life care, other factors must explain why clinicians still often do not use these techniques in caring for dying patients. There are many explanations of why patients, health care professionals, and health care organizations (HCOs) do not adequately deal with pain (Agency for Health Policy and Research, 1994; Bilkey, 1996; Starr, 1992; Atkinson and Davies, 1993; Cleeland, 1998; Martino, 1998; Ingham and Foley, 1998). The pain literature includes an interesting discussion of some of these possible explanations, such as:

- Health care professionals still lack adequate knowledge of pain assessment and treatment due to inadequate education and professional development;
- Health care professionals are concerned about legal and regulatory issues regarding the use of controlled substances in pain relief and the side effects of analgesics, such as tolerance, addiction, respiratory depression, loss of motor control, or constipation;
- Patients are reluctant to report pain because they don't want to distract doctors from their "real" diseases – because they think an increase in pain means a disease is getting worse; because they are concerned about the side-effects of analgesics, including addiction; because they think it is virtuous to put up with some pain; and because pain serves as an indicator of their health;
- HCOs do not provide adequate funding (or reimbursement) for pain assessment and treatment;
- Pain treatments are not always available (or accessible).

These explanations of medicine's failure to adequately deal with pain, while relevant, do not tell the whole story. Health care professionals have known about pain treatment techniques for many years: medical and nursing students learn about pain assessment and treatment in school; medical associations and pain initiatives have helped to remove some of the legal and regulatory barriers to proper pain management; and insurance companies and federal agencies fund treatments for pain (Martino, 1998). Furthermore, medical journals routinely publish new research on the importance of adequate pain control, and ethicists, patient advocates, medical associations, policy analysts, politicians, and lay people have demanded better palliative care in medicine. The word is getting out, but many people are still not getting the message. Why is this so? Why do these efforts at consciousness raising often fall on deaf ears?

One must go beyond the psychological, legal, social, and economic factors in the undertreatment of pain and explore cultural factors in medical practice in order to answer these questions. In this paper, I will place the culture of medicine on the examining table in order to develop a hypothesis that explains why pain is often undertreated. I will argue that modern medicine's scientific orientation plays a crucial role in the undertreatment of pain. Pain does not fit in well with the modern (scientific) medical paradigm. We will do a better job of treating pain only when medical culture becomes more humanistic in its orientation. To bring about this change, we need to revise medical education, research and practice to include more discussion of pain assessment and treatment, as well as the experience of pain.

2. PAIN AND SUFFERING

To get a clearer understanding of the issues, it will be useful to make several preliminary distinctions. The first distinction worth noting is between *pain* and *suffering*. These are two distinct notions: a person can be in pain without suffering and vice versa (Cassell, 1982). Long-distance runners may experience great pain during a race yet not suffer, and an artist who never sells a painting may suffer but not feel pain as a result of this failure. Although we recognize a distinction between pain and suffering, it is not easy to provide an uncontroversial account of this distinction, but I will offer one for the purpose of this essay. We tend to associate pain with specific, subjective experiences. Pain is primarily a kind of sensation or feeling that can occur at a specific time, be perceived in a specific location, or have a specific physiological basis, such as the pain of a burned finger, a sinus headache, a sprained ankle, and so on (Atkinson and Davies, 1993).

Suffering, on the other hand, is a much broader notion. Suffering can involve the awareness of something that threatens (or is perceived to threaten) the whole person (Cassell, 1982). A person can be viewed as a conscious being with a memory of the past, an awareness of the present, and plans and goals for the future. The whole person can be threatened by the existence of something that impedes future plans and goals. Recall the Greek myth of Sisyphus. The Gods punished Sisyphus for daring to be

God-like and made him roll a rock up a hill eternally. Although he may feel no pain, Sisyphus suffers because he is aware of his plight and his inability to achieve his goal (Camus, 1955). There are many ways that illness may bring about suffering. For example, a person may suffer as a result of prolonged and unremitting pain, since that person has the goal of relieving the pain but also because he has a memory of the pain, a present awareness of the pain, and an expectation that the pain will not go away. A person may also suffer as a result of dysfunction and disabilities caused by disease, such as incontinence, weakness, or paralysis.

Since the focus of this essay is pain, not suffering, I will not spend too much time discussing suffering. However, I would like to note that there is probably a gray area where we may have a very hard time distinguishing between pain and suffering, since pain often causes suffering and vice versa. A person who suffers as a result of unrequited love may start to feel pain, and a person whose pain is not relieved may suffer. These gray areas between pain and suffering show that pain is not simply a feeling caused by some specific neural pathway; there are also important psychosocial aspects of pain. I shall return to this point later.

Returning to the topic of pain, a second important distinction made by pain specialists is that between chronic and non-chronic (or acute) pain. Chronic pain is pain that either never ceases completely or recurs on a frequent basis for an indefinite period of time, such as the pain associated with arthritis, migraine headaches, or sickle cell anemia. If pain lasts for more than three months, it is usually considered chronic. Acute pain, on the other hand, ceases after some definite period of time, such as the pain from a broken finger, an ear infection, or labor.

A third distinction worth noting relates to the physical models of pain. Neurologists distinguish between nociceptive, neuropathic, and bone pain. In each of these types of pain, the sensation of pain is thought to result from stimulation of pain-sensitive nerve fibers. In nociceptive pain, tissue injury stimulates nerve fibers; in neuropathic pain, damaged or regenerated nerves spontaneously fire; in bone pain, damage to the bones stimulates nerve fibers. Of all of these types of pain, neuropathic pain is the least well understood. Classic examples of neuropathic pain include phantom limb pain and complex regional pain syndrome (Caudill et al., 1996).

Finally, it is useful to distinguish between pain in terminally ill patients and pain in patients who are not terminally ill. Patients who are terminally ill may suffer from chronic, acute, nociceptive, neuropathic, and bone pain (Caudill et al., 1996). This distinction is important because the side effects of analgesics, such as tolerance or addiction, may become less of a concern when patients are terminally ill, since there is less of a need to avoid side effects in these patients in order to prolong life.

Although this paper will focus on pain (in general), we need to be aware that different types of pain raise different medical, ethical and philosophical issues. For instance, since we often know the specific causes of nociceptive pain, it is often easier to assimilate this type of pain into the scientific approach to medicine, which emphasizes causal models of health and disease. We more readily believe that a person with a broken finger is in pain, but we have doubts about the pain experienced by people who display no signs of tissue damage.

3. THE GOALS OF MEDICINE

A close inspection of medical practice reveals that medicine has several, distinct goals. These goals can be divided into three categories, curative, palliative, and social. Curative goals include the aims of treating, curing, or preventing diseases in individual patients. Palliative goals include the aims of relieving pain and suffering through comfort, compassion, and care and promoting the overall well-being of patients. Social goals include the aims of promoting public health, knowledge advancement, social justice, or economic prosperity through medical practice.

The treatment of pain is only one of medicine's palliative goals. In medical practice, health care professionals must balance different goals in making health care decisions. Consider a hypothetical case of a 68-year-old man with inoperable, metastic colon cancer, diabetes mellitus, angina, and partial paralysis due to several recent strokes. Due to his illnesses, he also has reduced kidney, heart, and liver function. He is being treated for pain with morphine sulfate, taken orally. This medication, while highly effective in relieving pain, has some side effects, including physiological tolerance, reduced respiration, constipation, nausea, and drowsiness. The patient is already having difficulty with his bowel movements due to his bowel cancer. The patient would accept some pain in order to avoid constipation, drowsiness, and nausea. In order to manage the patient's pain, the clinician must balance this important goal against other clinical goals, such as maintaining adequate respiratory, bowel, liver, and kidney functions.

Other pain control decisions may involve a similar kind of clinical balancing act. For example, some kinds of pain relief can also interfere with labor. In deciding how to manage pain in labor and childbirth, the obstetrician and anesthesiologist must decide how to best provide pain relief while promoting the health of the mother and her child. Some sort of balancing also occurs when deciding how to manage non-terminal, chronic pain. The goal of pain relief must be weighed against other concerns, such as preventing narcotic addiction and excessive tolerance for pain medication (McCabe, 1997). Sometimes patients have difficulties with specific types of pain medications, such as Novocain or aspirin.

In order to understand the undertreatment of pain, it is therefore important that we realize that there are a variety of goals in medicine. Although sometimes pain is undertreated because it is simply not treated at all (as in many cases of circumcision in male infants), pain is often undertreated because health care professionals (and patients) place more weight on other goals. One of the objectives of this essay is to understand how and why pain relief sometimes takes a back seat in health care decisions. I will return to the question of balancing different goals shortly.

4. SCIENTIFIC MEDICINE

Earlier in this essay I characterized modern medicine as "scientific." Defining the term "scientific" is beyond the scope of this essay, but I will give a brief exposition of what I mean by this word. The following are some characteristics of professions or disciplines that we would call "scientific" (Popper, 1963; Merton, 1973; Ziman, 1984; Kitcher, 1993):

Methodology: members of the discipline attempt to follow procedures for developing knowledge that are similar to the procedures used in the physical sciences, such as testing, experimentation, quantitative measurement, and logical and statistical reasoning;

Language: Members of the discipline use specialized words and phrases (or jargon);

Theory structure: Members of the discipline attempt to articulate theories and concepts that can be understood in physical, chemical, or biological terms;

Expert knowledge: Members of the discipline are viewed as having expert knowledge as a result of their education, experience, and training;

Objectivity: Members of the discipline seek knowledge that is based on publicly observable, unbiased, and quantifiable evidence as opposed to knowledge that is private, biased, or not quantifiable.

Is modern medicine scientific? To answer this question, we need to distinguish between clinical medicine, public health, and medical research. Clinical medicine focuses on achieving curative and palliative goals for individual patients, public health aims at promoting the health of people in society, and medical research aims at developing medical knowledge concerning human populations. For the purposes of this essay, I will set aside the question of whether clinical research and public health are scientific and focus on clinical medicine. I shall argue that clinical medicine meets most of criteria listed above. Modern, clinical practice includes tests and experiments, quantitative measurements, and mathematical, logical, and statistical reasoning. Even treating a relatively simple problem, such as pneumonia, may require a battery of tests to eliminate possible diagnoses (e.g. lung cancer) or to promote health and safety (e.g. tuberculosis concerns). All of the health care professions employ a wide variety of specialized words and phrases, such as hemorrhage (bleeding), hydration (receiving water), cardiovascular (heart and circulation), and hypertension (high blood pressure). Medical jargon sounds like a foreign language to uninitiated lay people because it is a nomenclature that is based on specialized, scientific concepts and theories (Little, 1995).

Health care professionals are also regarded as having expert knowledge. Patients see doctors, in part, because they believe that doctors have some special, expert knowledge of health and disease (Little, 1995). Most of the key theories and concepts in medicine, such as the germ theory of disease, and the concept of thermal regulation, can be understood in physical, biological, or chemical terms. Finally, one might even argue that clinical medicine seeks objective knowledge, since clinical recommendations are based on publicly observable, unbiased, quantifiable phenomena. The evidenced-based movement in medical practice can be seen as an attempt to encourage clinicians to make judgments that are based on objective data and analysis, rather than on intuition or tradition (Little, 1995). It is no accident that medical schools require students to have a strong science background and that medical schools teach courses in the basic sciences and emphasize scientific reasoning in medicine; modern medicine is a highly scientific enterprise.

However, one might take issue with the argument that modern medicine is highly scientific. One might claim that while medicine aspires to be scientific, it will never be a *true* science like biology, chemistry, or physics. For example, Clouser and Zucker (1974) point out several features of clinical medicine that prevent it from being a true science, such as the centrality of human relationships, the importance of specific skills like surgery, the value-ladenness of medical concepts (e.g. health and disease), and the complexity of decision-making in clinical medicine. Other writers argue that medicine cannot be a science because it has practical goals (Munson, 1981; Little, 1995), it does not discover laws of nature (Schaffner, 1986, 1994), it uses analogical, case-based reasoning (Schaffner, 1986, 1994), or that it is applied to problems that often require urgent solutions (Caplan, 1986).

Although I do not have time to explore all of these interesting issues here, my overall assessment of this debate is that none of these arguments prove that medicine is not or cannot be highly scientific; at best, they prove that medicine operates with some constraints that prevent it from being as scientific as a "true" science like physics.

5. CLINICAL REASONING

Before exploring the place of pain treatment in scientific medicine, it is important to describe how clinicians (and other health care professionals) reason about medical problems, since pain treatment (and undertreatment) can be understood in this framework. We can think of clinical reasoning as a kind of decision-making that occurs during the processes of diagnosis, prognosis, and treatment (Albert et al., 1988; Sox et al., 1988). Arriving at a diagnosis in medicine is similar to proving a scientific hypothesis. The clinician begins with a problem or question based on the patient's current symptoms and case history (the initial data). She then develops a plausible guess (or hypothesis) about the patient's ailment(s) based on the initial data. In some cases, the clinician may not require additional data, but in other cases she tests this hypothesis through additional observations and controlled experiments (Resnik, 1995). She may also conduct tests in order to eliminate other possible hypotheses. If the tests disprove her initial hypothesis, then she develops other hypotheses and continues testing until she reaches a decision about what ails the patient (or a diagnosis). Due to constraints of time, money, and other resources, clinicians often do not achieve anything approaching diagnostic certainty; diagnoses are often highly probable, but fallible guesses (Gorovitz and MacIntyre, 1976; Sox et al., 1988).

Developing a prognosis is like making a prediction in science. The prediction can be based on the relevant evidence the clinician has at her disposal, such as the patient's diagnosis, symptoms, medical history, and statistical information. Since prognoses are usually based on diagnoses, they inherit diagnostic uncertainties (Sox et al., 1988). They can also be maligned by other uncertainties, such as unanticipated changes and developments in the patient and his illness, and difficulties in applying statistical generalizations to individual cases. There will always be patients who develop unexpected reactions to particular medications or interventions, patients who do not recover well from surgery, patients who develop additional complications or infections, as well as patients who do much better than expected and defy the odds. Thus, prognosis is even more fallible than diagnosis. Although predictions can be improved as clinicians obtain more evidence, clinicians and patients must often settle for rough guesses instead of reliable, exact prognoses (Gorovitz and MacIntyre, 1976).

Since treatment decisions are based on diagnoses and prognoses, they are infected by diagnostic and prognostic uncertainties. Since therapy aims at achieving particular goals for the patient, it also acquires the uncertainties relating to the proper balance of different goals. In recommending a course of treatment, a clinician must take into account the following considerations (factors or variables) which address the goals of treatment:

1. What treatments are available?
2. What are the medical benefits and risks of these different treatments?
3. What are the costs of the various treatments?
4. How painful or uncomfortable are the treatments?
5. What other information about the patient is relevant to making this decision?

In any particular case, there may be a wide variety of treatments available, including drugs, surgery, radiation, chemotherapy, dietary restrictions, exercise or physical therapy, as well as some combinations of different treatments or no treatment at all (Sox et al., 1988). Each of these different options may differ significantly in terms of medical risks and benefits, costs, pain, and discomfort. The treatment that is judged to be the safest and most effective may be very expensive or uncomfortable, the least painful treatment may not offer significant benefits, and so on. Furthermore, information about the patient, such as age, race, sex, risk factors, other treatments they are receiving, moral values, and economic status can significantly affect the choice of therapies. A therapy that would be recommended in a younger patient (such as a heart transplant) may not be recommended in an older patient; a therapy that is appropriate for most people (such as aspirin for a headache) would not be appropriate for a hemophiliac, an antibiotic appropriate for many people (such as acutane) would not be recommended for pregnant women, and so on.

In order to make a decision concerning a recommended course of treatment, therefore, a clinician must understand and assess all of these different considerations. Since clinicians must consider so many different variables at the same time, the reasoning is a highly complex type of cognitive juggling, and since different factors may be given different priorities in different cases, this reasoning is also situation-specific and informal (Clouser and Zucker, 1974.) No one has succeeded in completely formalizing the process of making a treatment decision, although some writers have attempted this task (Sox et al., 1988). Some formal methods, such as probability theory, statistics, decision theory, deductive logic, and computer programs can aid different parts of this process, but the process as a whole and the final decision still depends a great deal on human judgment, experience, and intuition (Little, 1995). A computer program may inform a clinician that a patient has a 90% chance of having deep vein thrombosis, given her signs and symptoms, but it is still the clinician, not the computer, who must make the diagnosis and accept responsibility for its implementation in therapy.

6. PAIN CONTROL AND CLINICAL REASONING

Given this overview of clinical reasoning, we can now understand how pain assessment and treatment fit (or fail to fit) into this decision-making process. Pain assessment can be viewed as a type of observation made by clinicians during diagnosis, prognosis, and treatment. Clinicians may consider questions such as:

Is the patient in pain? Where (in the body) is the pain? How severe is the pain? Does the pain stop or decrease? Does it increase? Does movement result in increased or decreased pain? What does the pain feel like? Is it dull? Does it burn or sting? Is it localized or general? Has the pain gotten better today? And so on.

Pain treatment can be viewed as a recommended course of therapy for managing, controlling, or eliminating pain. Thus, pain control becomes one additional consideration that a clinician must take into account when recommending a course of treatment, and it must be balanced against all of the other considerations mentioned above, such as medical benefits, risks, safety, efficacy, costs, discomfort, and so on (Atkinson and Davies, 1993; McCabe, 1997). Sometimes effective pain control will pose significant medical risks, such as decreased respiration or kidney function. Sometimes it will lead to adverse psychological problems, such as drug addiction. Sometimes it will result in discomfort, such as loss of motor control, nausea, or constipation. Although pain relief may often be the most important consideration from the patient's perspective, from the clinician's perspective it is usually just one more variable in a very complex case management plan (McCabe, 1997).

Given this portrait of the place of pain control in clinical decision-making, one can see how clinicians may sometimes decide to opt for less than adequate pain control in order to achieve other medical goals. Since clinicians are concerned about so many different medical variables, such as breathing, heart rate, blood flow, fluid levels, physical control, risk of infection, and so on, pain relief may sometimes get lost or be undervalued in the decision-making process. It is quite possible that many clinicians undertreat pain not because they don't care about pain (although this may also be the case), but because they give higher priority to a variety of medical considerations other than pain relief. For some, pain control may simply be the icing on the medical cake.

Giving a high priority to medical goals other than pain relief can be justified in many types of cases. For example, a pediatrician that treats a child's ear infection may prescribe ibuprofin to relieve pain and reduce the child's fever. While this drug may help the child to cope with pain of the ear infection, it probably will not completely eliminate the pain. A narcotic could completely relieve the child's pain, but it would also pose significant and unnecessary risks to the child's health. When the focus of treatment is curative rather than palliative, the benefits to the patient of complete pain relief are sometimes simply not worth the risks.

However, there are many types of cases in medicine where the goals of treatment are largely palliative rather than curative. When a patient has terminal ovarian cancer, the main goal should be providing comfort and pain control. Complete pain control may have adverse consequences for the patient's health, including death, but the benefits to the patient are worth the risks. A higher emphasis on pain control may also be appropriate in chronic pain cases as well, since pain may be the patient's primary symptom or complaint.

Thus, in many cases pain control should be given higher priority than it currently receives and in some cases it should be the primary focus of treatment. But a troubling question lingers: if health care professionals often should stress pain control, then why is pain control frequently inadequate? Why is pain so frequently undertreated even when there are good reasons for relieving pain? In the introduction to this essay I briefly mentioned some answers to these questions, but I will now put forward an explanation that should be considered in more depth: pain is often undertreated because it does not fit in well with the scientific approach to medicine.

7. PAIN AND SCIENTIFIC MEDICINE

Earlier in this paper, I discussed reasons why modern medicine is a scientific discipline even though it may not be a *true* science. The scientific approach to medicine has proved to be very useful in achieving medicine's curative and social goals, but it may be detrimental to achieving palliative goals, such as pain control. There are several reasons why pain does not fit the scientific approach to medicine. The *first* is that it does not easily succumb to objective tests, measurements, or diagnostic procedures. You cannot use X-rays, CT-scans, sonograms, or biopsies to observe pain. You cannot measure pain in the same way you can measure body temperature, pulse, blood pressure, blood oxygen levels, or even brain activity. Although pain can have various physiological effects, such as increased pulse or blood pressure, or behavioral manifestations, such as wincing, screaming, or the gnashing of teeth, or even psychological effects, such as depression, to get a good indication of pain health care professionals must rely on first-person (subjective) reports (Atkinson and Davies, 1993). Although pain is usually associated with tissue damage and other physiological causes, the reason we care about treating pain is that pain is a subjective experience (sensation or feeling) that most people prefer to avoid. Although we all know what pain feels like, we will never be able to experience someone else's pain. Pain is a private experience.

We can no more experience another person's pain than we can experience their joy, their love of Mozart, their aversion to anchovies, or their suffering.

In response to this problem, pain specialists have developed elaborate techniques and tools for pain assessment. In using these techniques, health care professionals (often nurses) request patients to classify pain according to various characteristics, such as quality (dull or stinging), localization (local or general), location, duration, intensity, and frequency. Patients may rate their pain on a scale of 1 to 10 and they may also keep a pain diary to record how various treatments have affected their pain. Physiological responses, such as heart rate and blood pressure, can also be used in pain assessment. Many people who have developed these pain assessment tools have even recommended that pain be viewed as a fifth vital sign (Agency for Health Policy and Research, 1994; Caudill, 1994; Kerns et al., 1985; Atkinson and Davies, 1993; World Health Organization, 1990).

While I think these methods are important clinical tools and I would not dissuade health care professionals from using whatever means they may have at their disposal to assess pain, these techniques do not transform pain into a publicly observable phenomena. Pain is still a private experience. What I say to you about my pain is publicly observable, but what I feel is not. What I write in a pain journal is publicly observable, but my pain is not. The assessment tools are merely elaborate, well-organized ways of reporting private experiences.

These assessment techniques also do not make pain quantifiable in any meaningful way. In order to quantify measurements, the measurements must be commensurable (comparable). We can quantify height because we can compare two different structures in terms of a common scale. We can quantify height by using an absolute scale, such as a ruler, or a relative one, such as an arrangement of structures in terms of the relation "higher than." But we cannot do this with pain, at least not in any definite way. Since pain is private, we cannot compare our pain against a public scale, such as a yardstick. And although each person might be able to use a relative scale to assess his own pain, e.g., my sprained foot hurts twice as much as that sore thumb I had last month, we cannot use this kind of scale to make interpersonal comparisons of pain. We have no way of knowing whether my sprained ankle hurts more than your sprained ankle. Thus, the mere act of attaching numbers to personal reports of pain does not make pain quantifiable. The numbers, while perhaps useful, are illusory.

A second reason why pain does not fit the scientific model is that the physiological causes of pain are often not known or well understood. As I mentioned earlier, neuropathic pain is still not well understood. When patients report pain and clinicians do not know the physiological causes of the pain, there is a tendency to view the pain as psychosomatic or fraudulent (Bilkey, 1996). Many chronic pain patients with neuropathic pain have been accused of faking their pain in order to obtain workers' compensation or file health insurance claims. This is similar to what happens to patients who suffer from diseases that are poorly understood, such as chronic fatigue syndrome. When we don't know the physiological basis of a medical condition, we frequently tend to view it as psychosomatic or not "real."

Additionally, pain often has strong psychological, cultural, and social components (Gatchel and Turk, 1996; Caudill, 1994; Atkinson and Davies, 1993). For example, injuries produce different sensations of pain in different people and different people seem to have different tolerances for pain. Pain causes depression and stress in some people but not in others. Some patients can use biofeedback and meditation to control pain; others cannot. Some cultures (and religions) view some types of pain as ennobling ("pain is good for you" or "no pain, no gain"); others view pain as a curse. Some cultures (and religions) expect people to put up with a great deal of pain ("grin and bear it" or "bite the bullet"); others do not. Finally, as I noted earlier, various types of suffering may cause pain.

Since psychosocial factors can influence our experience of pain, pain judgments are also inherently biased. They are more like judgments of taste or feeling than unbiased reports. A judgment can be said to be "biased" if it is shaped by personal beliefs, interests and assumptions and philosophical, religious, and ideological assumptions. For example, General Motors' judgment about the value of their new mini-van is biased because it is shaped by the company's interest in making money; a mother's assessment of her daughter's intelligence is biased because it is shaped by her beliefs about her daughter. Psychosocial factors can shape our judgments about the severity of pain, its duration, and so on.

Since the physiological causes of pain are often not well known or understood, it is often difficult to explain pain in terms of currently accepted theories from the "true" sciences of biology, chemistry, and physics. Indeed, this problem is not unique to pain, since other psychosocial phenomena, such as consciousness, intelligence, color perception, creativity, art, and language, also cannot be explained in terms of currently accepted theories from the "true" sciences. Viewed in this way, the problem of explaining pain is part of the larger philosophical/scientific project of understanding the human mind and human behavior. Thus, the solution to a key problem in the philosophy of medicine – understanding pain – may depend on our ability to set psychology and the human sciences on a scientific footing. Although many scholars have argued that psychology and the social sciences cannot be reduced to natural sciences, we do not yet have a satisfactory and uncontroversial resolution to this debate (Rosenberg, 1995; Jaquette, 1994). I will not explore these larger issues here.

A third reason why pain does not fit the scientific conception of medicine is that health care professionals have not developed a specialized language for talking about pain. Virtually every surgical procedure, every drug, every anatomical feature, and every disease has its own special name based on scientific theories and concepts. Furthermore, it is surprising how little some health care professionals actually talk about pain. One has only to read the medical literature, review a medical record, or attend a medical conference to see that most of the words refer to medical phenomena other than pain. Perhaps pain is not talked about because the word "pain" is a term from the vernacular. Since professionals are sometimes inclined to use jargon and technical terms, one might cynically suggest that developing some new, arcane, "scientific" words to describe pain would elevate pain's place in medical discussions. Since language often reflects our assumptions, theories, biases, and commitments, however, an attempt to reform medical language may not prove to be ultimately successful. People tend to describe those things they know and care about. Eskimos have a special terminology for snow; health care professionals have special terminology for human anatomy and physiology. Health care professionals will not develop a special terminology for pain until they place more value on the treatment of pain.

The final reason why pain does not fit the scientific approach to medicine is that it does not conform to the model of expert knowledge. To be an expert, one must have knowledge, experience, judgment, or skill that lay people lack (Hardwig, 1994). Lay people depend on experts to make judgments, decisions, and recommendations because they trust that the experts are better qualified to make these judgments, decisions, and recommendations. Since there are no special scientific tests for detecting pain and very little jargon for classifying it, pain does not fit the model of expert knowledge. Our knowledge of pain is more like common opinion or folk wisdom than scientific belief. Now it is true that neurologists, anesthesiologists, pharmacologists, psychologists, and pain specialists have expert knowledge about the physiological basis of pain and the treatment of pain. But when it comes to experience of pain, lay people know just about as much about pain as these experts. This is an interesting twist for health care professionals, who usually have much more medical knowledge than their patients. When it comes to their own pain, patients have the upper hand.

8. CONCLUSION: ADVOCATING PAIN

To sum up the argument so far, I have characterized modern medicine as a scientific discipline, and I have argued that pain does not fit in well with this approach to health care. Pain is an enigma because it is cannot be measured or observed by means of objective tests, its physiological basis is often understood poorly, it lacks a specialized terminology, and it does not fit the model of expert knowledge. Since clinicians are trained in scientific methods, techniques, theories, and concepts, it is often difficult for them to deal with, acknowledge, understand, and talk about pain. Since pain treatment must compete against other considerations in a management plan for a patient, it may sometimes be under-valued in the complex process of deciding what is best for a patient. Other medical considerations tend to speak more clearly and forcefully; it is often easier for clinicians to grasp the significance of a low blood oxygen level or elevated temperature than it is for them to understand the significance of pain. It is much easier to ignore someone's pain than it is to ignore a freely bleeding wound or persistent cough. It is easier to undertreat pain than it is to undertreat diabetes.

If my hypothesis is correct, then what are its implications? First, the hypothesis helps us to understand and explain why pain continues to be undertreated despite the recent successes of the palliative care movement. Second, since many of the arguments examined in this essay also apply to other phenomena that do not conform with the scientific approach, such as suffering, it may allow us to understand why modern medicine has difficulty dealing with these phenomena. Third, the hypothesis implies that the problem of the undertreatment of pain goes much deeper than removing legal/regulatory barriers to pain treatment or providing sufficient reimbursement for pain medications. The problem cuts to the very heart of modern medicine, which emphasizes scientific methods to achieve curative and social goals.

Some advocates for better palliative care argue that the entire discipline of medicine needs to become more humanistic (Little, 1995). I agree with this position, to a certain extent. However, I am also realistic. The scientific approach to medicine has been enormously successful and is supported by several centuries of medical lore and tradition. No one can (or should) expect medicine to become more humanistic in the next decade or the next generation. However, I think there are some things that can done which would help to address the problem of the undertreamtent of pain.

First, pain control should have a more prominent place in medical education (Foley, 1997; AMA, 1997; McCabe, 1997; Martino, 1998). Students in the health care professions need to learn more about assessment and treatment as well as how pain affects patients and their families. Health care professionals also need to know a bit more about the experience of pain. I am not suggesting that teachers should make students feel pain, but it might not be a bad idea to have students spend more time discussing pain with people who are experiencing it. Second, there should be more research on pain assessment and pain treatment (McCabe, 1997). We need to develop analgesics and surgical techniques that do not have some of the side effects that make clinicians hesitant to emphasize pain control. Since western medicine has had trouble dealing with pain, we should also conduct more research on non-western approaches to pain control, such as acupuncture or meditation. Third, we need to advocate for pain in as many ways as we can. To advocate literally means "to speak for." To advocate for pain, we need to talk about it more often and more seriously. Health care professionals should discuss pain with their patients and with each other. Conferences about management plans for patients should include more discussion of pain. The voice of pain needs to be heard, not locked away in a hospital room or nursing home.

If clinicians hear the voice of pain and respond to it, they may reduce the demand for physician-assisted suicide. This type of change in the culture of medicine could help to undercut some of the key arguments for this practice. However, if this change never occurs or it comes about very slowly, then proponents of physician-assisted suicide could argue that patients need to have this option available because their pleas for pain control and palliation may fall on deaf ears. Until the culture of medicine transforms, there will be a need for physician-assisted suicide to relieve pain and suffering. Recognizing the need to advocate for pain is thus a double-edged sword that could be wielded by either side of the physician-assisted suicide debate. These reflections suggest that this aspect of the controversy penetrates well beyond empirical questions about techniques for pain control and palliation and strikes at the heart of current medical practice. Coming to some acceptable resolution of the physician-assisted suicide debate therefore requires us to assess, critique, and change the culture of medicine.

Acknowledgments: The author would like to thank Loretta M. Kopelman, John Moskop, Ken De Ville, Daniel Klein, and Ann Jacobs for helpful discussions and comments.

Brody School of Medicine at East Carolina University
Greenville, North Carolina

NOTES

[1] Chronic pain often poses a whole range of ethical and medical issues, since patients with chronic pain can develop high tolerances for pain medications, can become addicted, can become depressed, or can develop a psychological condition known as chronic pain syndrome (Caudill, 1994).

[2] Medicine may be best characterized as a type of applied science like engineering or computer science. Engineers, like health care professionals, have to engage in relationships with clients and the public; they have to develop special skills, such as model building and drafting; they employ value-laden concepts (e.g., safety and risk), they do not discover laws of nature, and they must make complex decisions that consider and assess many different variables. Engineers also have practical goals (e.g., designing bridges that don't fall down), they use analogical reasoning that refers to cases and particular problem-solutions, and they must solve problems based on specific time-constraints (Whitbeck, 1995).

The second objection to my position admits that modern medicine is highly scientific but maintains that it *ought* not to be as scientific as it (regrettably) is. One might argue that the scientific approach to medicine ignores important human values and concerns, such as pain, suffering, autonomy, quality of life, and justice, and that it creates health care professionals (especially doctors) who are incompassionate, uncaring people. Medicine should become less scientific and more humanistic, one might argue (Little, 1995; Pellegrino and Thomasma, 1981).

To a certain extent I agree with this line of reasoning; I also suspect that medicine has become excessively scientific. But I balk at claiming that medical practice should err in the other direction. One need look no further than the recent history of medicine (e.g., snake oil salesmen) or its current history (e.g., food and vitamin supplements) to see the importance of preventing quackery and deception. Since medicine deals with issues that are of significant moral concern, such as matters of life and death and human health, it is important to develop reliable, unbiased knowledge and expertise in medicine. People trust doctors with their lives and health, and they expect that they will receive competent, professional care when they request it (Pellegrino and Thomasma, 1993). In order to insure that health care meets high standards of quality, safety, competence, and reliability, scientific methods, concepts, and theories should play an important role in medical education, research, public health, and clinical decision-making.

REFERENCES

Agency for Health Policy and Research: 1994, *Clinical Practice Guideline: Management of Cancer Pain*, U.S. Department of Health and Human Services Rockville, MD.

Albert, D., Munson, R., Resnik, M.: 1988, *Reasoning in Medicine*, Johns Hopkins University Press, Baltimore.

AMA, Council on Scientific Affairs: 1997, 'Good care of the dying patient', *Journal of the American Medical Association* 275 (6), 474–478.

Atkinson, R. and Davies, G.: 1993, 'Issues in pain management', in D. Clark (ed.) *The Future of Palliative Care*, Open University Press, Buckingham, pp.148–166.

Beauchamp, T. and Childress, J.: 1994, *Principles of Biomedical Ethics*, 4th edition, Oxford University Press, New York.

Bilkey, W.: 1996, 'Confusion, fear, and chauvinism: perspectives on the medical sociology of chronic pain', *Perspectives in Biology and Medicine* 39 (2), 270–280.

Byock, I.: 1997, *Dying Well*, Riverhead Books, New York.

Camus, A.: 1955, *The Myth of Sisyphus*, Vintage Books, New York.

Caplan A.: 1986, 'Exemplary reasoning? A comment on theory structure in Biomedicine', *Journal of Medicine and Philosophy* 11, 93–105.

Cassell, E.: 1982, 'The nature of suffering and the goals of medicine', *New England Journal of Medicine* 306, 639–645.

Caudill, M.: 1994, *Managing Pain Before it Manages You*, Guilford Press, New York.

Cleeland, C.: 1998, 'Undertreatment of cancer pain in elderly patients', *Journal of the American Medical Association* 279 (23), 1914–1915.

Cleeland, C. et al.: 1994, 'Pain and its treatment in outpatients with metastatic cancer', *New England Journal of Medicine* 330, 592–596.

Clouser, K. and Zucker, A.: 1974, 'Medicine as an art: an initial exploration', *Texas Reports on Biology and Medicine* 2, 267–274.

Culver, C. and Gert, B.: 1982, *Philosophy in Medicine*, Oxford University Press, New York.

Cupples, S.: 1992, 'Pain as a hurtful experience: a philosophical analysis and implications for nursing care', *Nursing Forum* 27 (1), 5–11.

DeShano, C.: 1997, 'Michigan moves toward better pain management', *Michigan Medicine* 96 (1), 16–21.

Emanuel, E., Daniels, E., Fairclough, D., Clarridge, B.: 1998, 'The practice of euthanasia and physician-assisted suicide in the United States', *Journal of the American Medical Association* 280, 507–513.

Emanuel, L.: 1998, 'Facing requests for physician-assisted suicide', *Journal of the American Medical Association* 280, 643–647.

Foley, K.: 1997, 'Competent care for the dying instead of physician-assisted suicide', *New England Journal of Medicine* 336 (1), 54–58.

Gatchell, R. and Turk, D.: 1996, *Psychological Approaches to Pain Management*, Guilford Press, New York.

Goldstein, N.: 1997, 'Inadequate pain management: a suicidogen', *Journal of Clinical Pharmacology* 37 (1), 1–3.

Gorovitz, S. and MacIntyre, A.: 1976, 'Towards a theory of medical fallibility', *Journal of Medicine and Philosophy* 1, 51–71.

Hardwig, J.: 1994, 'Toward an ethics of expertise', in D. Wueste (ed.) *Professional Ethics and Social Responsibility*, Rowman and Littlefield, Lanham, MD, 83–101.

Harrold, J. and Lynn, J.: 1998, *A Good Dying*. New York: The Haworth Press.

Harvey, W.: 1993, *On the Motion of the Heart and Blood in Animals*, R Willis (trans.), Prometheus Books, Buffalo.

Hill, C.: 1995, 'When will adequate pain control be the norm?', *Journal of the American Medical Association* 274, 1881–1882.

Horgan J.: 1997, 'Seeking a better way to die', *Scientific American* 276 (5), 100–105.

Ingham, J. and Foley, K.: 1998, 'Pain and the barriers to its relief at the end-of-life: a lesson for improving end-of-life care', *The Hospice Journal* 13 (1 & 2), 89–100.

Jaquette, D.: 1994, *Philosophy of Mind*, Prentice-Hall, Englewood Cliffs, NJ.

Jost, T.: 1998, 'Public financing of pain management: leaky umbrellas and ragged safety nets', *Journal of Law, Medicine, and Ethics* 26, 290–307.

Kerns, R., Turk, D., Rudy, T.: 1985, 'The West Haven-Yale multidimensional pain inventory', *Pain* 23, 345–356.

Kitcher, P.: 1993, *The Advancement of Science*, Oxford University Press, New York.

Little, M.: 1995, *Humane Medicine*, Cambridge University Press, Cambridge.

Lynn, J. and Wilkinson, A.: 1998, 'Quality end-of-life care: the case for a Medicaring demonstration', *The Hospice Journal* 13 (1 & 2), 151–163.

Martino, A.: 1998, 'In search of a new ethic for treating patients with chronic pain: what can medical boards do?', *Journal of Law, Medicine, and Ethics* 26, 332–349.

McCabe, M.: 1997, 'Ethical issues in pain management', *The Hospice Journal* 12 (2), 25–32.

McGivney, W. and Crooks, G.: 1984, 'The care of patients with severe chronic pain in terminal illness', *Journal of the American Medical Association* 25, 1182–1188.

Meadows, J.: 1992, *The Great Scientists*, Oxford University Press, New York.

Merton, R. 1973. *The Sociology of Science*. University of Chicago Press, Chicago.

Munson, R.: 1981, 'Why medicine cannot be a science', *Journal of Medicine and Philosophy* 6, 183–208.

Ng, B., Dimsdale, J., Sharagg, G., Deutsch, R.: 1996, 'Ethnic differences in analgesic consumption for postoperative pain', *Psychosomatic Medicine* 58, 125–129.

Pellegrino, E. and Thomasma, D.: 1981, *A Philosophical Basis of Medical Practice*, Oxford University Press, New York.

Pellegrino, E. and Thomasma, D.: 1993, *The Virtues in Medical Practice*. Oxford University Press, New York.

Popper, K.: 1963, *Conjectures and Refutations*. Harper and Rower, New York.

Porter, R.: 1997, *The Greatest Benefit of Mankind*, WW Norton, New York.

Quill, T., Cassell, C., Meier, D.: 1992, 'Care of the hopelessly ill: proposed clinical criteria for physician-assisted suicide', *New England Journal of Medicine* 327, 1380–1384.

Quill, T., Lo, B., Brock, D.: 1997, 'Palliative options of last resort', *Journal of the American Medical Association* 278, 2099–2104.

Resnik, D.: 1995, 'To test or not to test: a clinical dilemma', *Theoretical Medicine* 16, 1–12.

Rollin, B.: 1997, 'Pain and ideology in human a veterinary medicine', *Seminars in Veterinary Medicine and Surgery* 12 (2), 56–60.

Rosenberg, A.: 1995, *Philosophy of Social Science*, 2nd edition, Westview *Press*, Boulder, CO.

Schaffner, K.: 1994, *Discovery and Explanation in Biology and Medicine*, University of Chicago Press, Chicago.

Schaffner, K.: 1986, 'Exemplary reasoning about biological models and diseases: a relation between the philosophy of medicine and the philosophy of science', *Journal of Medicine and Philosophy* 11, 63–80.

Singer, P. and Siegler, M.: 1990, 'Euthanasia: a critique', *New England Journal of Medicine* 322, 1881–1883.

Sox, H., Blatt, M., Higgins, M., Marton, K.: 1988, *Medical Decision Making*. Butterworths, Boston.

Starr, S.: 1992, 'The politics of pain: a new attitude toward treatment', *Drug Topics* 136 (18), 60–70.

SUPPORT Principal Investigators: 1997, 'A controlled trial to improve care for seriously ill hospitalized patients', *Journal of the American Medical Association* 274 (20), 1591–1598.

Sullivan, M., Rapp, S., Fitzgibbon, D., Chapman, C.: 1997, 'Pain and the choice to hasten death in patients with painful metastatic cancer', *Journal of Palliative Care* 13 (3), 18–28.

Todd, K., Samaria, N., Hoffman, J.: 1993, 'Ethnicity as a risk factor for inadequate emergency department analgesia', *Journal of the American Medical Association* 269, 1537–1539.

Whitbeck, C.: 1995, 'Teaching ethics to scientists and engineers: moral agents and moral problems', *Science and Engineering Ethics* 1, 299–308.

World Health Organization: 1990, *Cancer Pain Relief and Palliative Care*. World Health Organization, Geneva.

Ziman, J.: 1984, *An Introduction to Science Studies*, Cambridge University Press, Cambridge.

STEVEN H. MILES

MANAGED HEALTH CARE AT THE END OF LIFE[1]

1. INTRODUCTION

The vast majority of discussion regarding physician-assisted suicide has implicitly assumed the existence of a private and traditional physician–patient relationship. Jurisprudential, legislative and philosophical debates have, for the most part, been based on the culture of the dyadic doctor–patient relationship in which physician and patient together decide what course of treatments would be most appropriate. That paradigm can no longer be assumed. It is clear that the so-called managed care revolution is irrevocably transforming the delivery of health care in this country. Health care payors – insurance companies, managed care organizations (MCOs), and the government – are increasingly and dramatically playing a larger role in health care management to monitor care and to contain costs. They do so largely by influencing, channeling, and limiting the decision-making prerogatives of physicians. Moreover, the growth of managed care has been so dramatic and rapid that in a relatively short time the majority of U.S. citizens are likely to receive their care from some form of managed care plan. Thus, physician-assisted suicide, if it is practiced, is likely to be practiced in a managed care culture.

A full discussion of physician-assisted suicide and its advisability must take account of these fundamentally changed circumstances in the new practice culture of managed care. A few authors have noted the significance of the managed care context for the policy decisions that must be made regarding physician-assisted suicide. John La Puma, for example, has suggested that physician-assisted suicide and managed care is "a match made in hell" (La Puma, 1997). Cathleen Kaveny observes that most of the most prominent and sympathetic vignettes of physician-assisted suicide have involved individuals who have died on their "own terms," an option she suggests may not be possible in the practice context of managed care (Kaveny, 1998). Instead, cost-conscious measures imposed by managers and implemented by physicians threaten to influence both patient and physician decision making. Similarly, Susan

Loretta M. Kopelman and Kenneth A. De Ville (eds.), Physician-Assisted Suicide, 149–167.
© 2001 *Kluwer Academic Publishers. Printed in Great Britain.*

Wolf is skeptical that states can effectively frame safeguards against assisted suicide abuse in a medical culture dominated by managed care. Physician decision making is likely to be affected in a number of important ways. As importantly, the "systemic neglect" that may be the consequence of some managed care approaches might play a major and baneful role in patients' decisions to pursue the assisted suicide option (Wolf, 1996).

Commentators on physician-assisted suicide, both pro and con, have long understood that the policy debate on physician-assisted suicide must include a consideration of the realities of end-of-life care. This essay sketches the realities of end-of-life care in the managed care context in the hope of providing a clearer view of the practice culture in which legislatures, judges, patients and physicians will make what are life-and-death decisions about physician-assisted suicide. It: 1) outlines major issues for managed end-of-life care, 2) examines the epidemiology of end-of-life care in MCOs especially in relation to U.S. health policy, and 3) examines the research about how well managed end-of-life care serves people using paradigmatic patterns of end-of-life care. Finally, it will discuss the implications of this analysis for improving managed end-of-life care.

I define an MCO as an entity that sells health insurance and administers the provision of health care. An MCO holds a diverse set of health care providers accountable for providing specified health services (a benefit set) to a defined population (plan members) for a defined set of resources (premiums). This definition includes staff–model health maintenance organizations (HMOs) as well as preferred-provider plans where financial risks hold clinicians financially accountable for part of the cost of providing services to members. This simultaneous accountability of clinicians to members and resources make cost-containment an explicit value in managed health care and distinguishes managed care from fee-for-service reimbursement in which the financing system and clinical decisions are separated. Health care for the last year of life accounts for 10% of U.S. health care spending (Scitovsky, 1994).

"End-of-life care" broadly includes unsuccessful aggressive attempts to prolong life as well as purely palliative treatments. This paper focuses on the delivery system for end-of-life care rather than limiting its scope to persons who have chosen to forgo life-sustaining treatments.

The relative merits of managed health care versus fee-for-service reimbursement are incompletely understood. Fee-for-service allows for a purer form of physician advocacy for treatment but fails by fragmenting health care delivery, promoting poor coordination between medical and social services and between hospital and community-based health care, incentivizing overtreatment, and having poor quality assurance for services as basic as pain control.

MCOs potentially could improve the coordination of referrals among the diverse health care providers engaged in a patient's end-of-life care (Miles et al., 1995). A well-designed network of hospital, home care, hospice, and nursing home care services would not have dysfunctional incentives to needlessly base end-of-life health care in the hospital. For example, an MCO could decrease the incentive to underuse hospice care by a fee-for-service oncologist who fears losing a "paying customer." MCOs, unlike individual clinicians, must develop, accept, and disseminate advance directives (Fade and Kaplan, 1995). An MCO has demonstrated its ability to successfully recruit durable powers of attorney for end-of-life decision making (Rubin et al., 1994). Though cost containment seems to encourage MCOs to promote living wills, one study found that AIDS patients at an academic health center were more likely to have living wills than HMO patients (Haas et al., 1993). MCO information systems could promote better interfacility communication of treatment plans as patients move between clinics, hospitals, home care, hospices and nursing homes (Sachs et al., 1991; Danis et al., 1991, Morrison and Meir, 1995). MCOs often serve very large populations and have large amounts of capital that can support innovative programs, for example, home hospice programs for poor persons without informal caregivers (Pawling-Kaplan and O'Connor, 1989; Brenner, 1997).

MCOs are not trusted. Cost-containment pressures may compromise physician advocacy, especially for vulnerable or stigmatized persons who need costly health care. Some fear that this will lead to withholding beneficial care or create an incentive for physician-assisted suicide (Wolf, 1997; Sulmasy, 1995). It is not known whether this danger can be offset by risk-adjusted capitation (see below), quality promotion incentives, public disclosure of outcomes, ombudsmen offices, or diluting the financial risk that is brought to bear on clinicians (Hillman, 1995). Many fear that information systems threaten patient confidentiality and will be used for insurance or employment discrimination (Gostin et al., 1993). Public distrust may improve with greater public accountability, with reforms to secure access to insurance, and with studies showing that managed care delivers good quality outcomes (Mechanic and Schilesinger, 1996).

The quality of end-of-life care by MCOs parallels changes in the U.S. health care system with regard to end-of-life care and the overall performance of MCOs. The Institute of Medicine and the American Board of Internal Medicine (Field and Cassel, 1997) recently discussed features of the American health care system that adversely affect end-of-life care. Absent universal health insurance, an MCO benefits by shifting a costly dying patient to another insurer. MCOs are unlikely to make up for inadequate clinical training in end-of-life care or to provide end-of-life services that consumers do not demand until overwhelmed by care-giving or disability (Dossetor and MacDonald, 1994; Institute of Medicine, 1997).

Employers, the voluntary purchasers of health care, largely determine the services offered by MCOs. The Employment Retirement Income Security Act (ERISA) allows "self-insured" employers to define insurance benefits virtually unencumbered by state insurance mandates or consumer preferences (Employment Retirement Income Security Act of 1974). Thus, MCOs are the employers' agents for selling health care benefits and providing health care services.

- A recent federal ERISA reform prevents insurers from denying coverage for preexisting conditions to persons who change jobs so long as they remain continuously insured during the job change (Health Insurance Portability and Accountability Act). This provision would protect an HIV-infected person with a history of AIDS who switched to a new job if the subsequent employer offered HIV coverage to other comparable employees. But, it does not require a new employer to equal the previous employer's coverage nor would it prevent the second employer from deciding to discontinue extended AIDS treatment for all employees.
- ERISA was recently amended to require employers' health plans to have the same total dollar limit for mental illnesses as for physical conditions (Frank et al., 1997). This would seem to improve insurance for the common mental illnesses, like depression, that occur in terminally ill persons. The limited life span of terminally ill persons makes it unlikely that they would be able to use anywhere near the same amount of mental health services as physical health services. Furthermore, this reform does not bar an MCO from imposing higher copays or deductibles for mental health services than for physical

health services, and thus leaves intact the considerable out-of-pocket price barriers to obtaining mental health services.

2. EMPIRICAL RESEARCH OF MANAGED END-OF-LIFE CARE

There are many reasons why end-of-life care by MCOs is uncharted.

- First, "end-of-life care" is not an easily defined episode of treatment. It occurs in the course of many illnesses (cancer, heart disease, and trauma, etc.). It takes place in diverse settings including hospitals, intensive care units, nursing homes, home care programs, and primary care and specialty clinics. It lasts varying lengths of time from sudden catastrophic strokes or fatal trauma to the indolent course of Alzheimer's disease.
- Second, MCOs provide relatively little end-of-life care. They mainly provide employer-based insurance for working people with low death rates. Six percent of persons over 65 years old die each year, accounting for 69% of U.S. deaths (Emanuel, E. and Emanuel, L, 1994). MCOs enroll about 10% of Medicare patients (Lamphere, et al., 1997), though the proportion of Medicare enrollees in any given plan varies widely. The Kaiser plans in southern California have 250,000 persons over age 65 (Snow, 1996). Furthermore, MCO Medicare enrollees have a 20% lower death rate than Medicare fee-for-service members (Riley et al., 1991). Data show how increasing enrollment and an increasing percentage of Medicare enrollees may affect the amount of end-of-life care in MCOs. Little is written about end-of-life care for the rapidly increasing Medicaid managed care population (Rowland and Hanson, 1996).
- Third, research on end-of-life care by MCOs is difficult to assess. There is no mandatory or universal reporting of the amount, characteristics, or quality of end-of-life care. Quality standards for end-of-life care are in their methodological infancy (Institute of Medicine, 1997; Donaldson, 1996; Wenger and Rothenberg, 1996). Voluntarily published corporate research often showcases "model" results (Rennie, 1997; Shimm and Spece, 1991; Barnes and Bero, 1996) and thus may be unrepresentative, ungeneralizable, or biased.
- The major issues for managed end-of-life care are: 1) enrollment (or disenrollment) of persons at high risk of needing end-of-life care, 2) the availability of insurance for needed services, and 3) the quality of

care. Given the diversity of end-of-life care, it is helpful to consider these issues as they arise in paradigmatic diseases. These are: 1) indolent progressive diseases (e.g., AIDS or Alzheimer's disease), 2) subacute terminal illnesses (e.g., many cancers), and 3) acute catastrophic deaths (e.g., trauma or fatal heart attacks) (Lynn, 1997).

3. INDOLENT PROGRESSIVE DISEASES: AIDS

Indolent progressive diseases, like AIDS or Alzheimer's disease, are those in which persons are seriously chronically ill and dying for several years. Such diseases exemplify the elusive and shifting transition from curative treatment, to minimizing treatment burdens, to purely palliative care. Such a course is a common trajectory to death. A health care system that could meet the needs of these patients could meet the needs of patients dying of subacute and progressive "terminal" illnesses.

Being the longest terminal course, indolent progressive illness is the most costly form of end-of-life care (Riley et al., 1987; Christakis and Escarce, 1996). There is reason to fear that MCOs may deny insurance to persons with AIDS or develop marketing strategies to avoid enrollees at risk of such deaths. As persons with AIDS or early dementia change jobs or retire because of disability or to move near caregivers, insurers have opportunities to discontinue coverage or prevent enrolling such persons both to decrease the costs of providing health care and to offer more competitive premiums to employers who purchase MCO health plans for healthier persons.

Two reforms have been proposed to compensate for dysfunctional incentives that lead insurers to charge prohibitively high premiums for persons with AIDS or to seek members less likely to need this form of end-of-life health care. In community-rating, premiums are the same regardless of risk of needing more health care. This creates higher premiums for the healthy and has an implicitly communitarian ethic about the collective vulnerability of all persons to illness and the shared responsibility for assuring access to health care (Daniels, 1990). Risk-adjusted reimbursement is when a public payer compensates health plans in proportion to their exposure to the higher costs of members with a severe chronic disease and thus decreases the disincentive for enrolling such persons" (Padgug, 1995). Similarly, an MCO may supplement the standard capitation to its providers who undertake the care of such patients to prevent a high-cost patient from being under-served by financially at-risk providers. Risk-adjusting for chronic, progressive disease is extremely complex and experimental (Kahn et al., 1995). It is affected by the varying severity of diseases and the changing costs of clinical needs at each stage. It changes as new therapies are introduced at the beginning, middle, and late stages of disease (Scitovsky et al., 1990). For example, protease inhibitors change the cost of treating persons with early AIDS; the use of total parenteral nutrition changes the cost of late-stage disease. If protease inhibitors prolong life, the number of persons with AIDS in the treated population increases as the mortality rate falls.

Many MCOs use case management to control the costs of treating persons with AIDS. These programs: 1) stratify patients according to severity of illness or need; 2) integrate medical and mental health care, and social work, hospice, volunteer, and home care services, to control use of costly services like hospitalization, nursing home care, or parenteral nutrition; 3) coordinate public and private resources; and 4) develop practice guidelines (Sowell and Meadows, 1994; Taravella, 1988; Yox, 1990; Japsen, 1994; Sowell, 1995; Sowell and Griere, 1995; Sonsel, 1989; Ryndes, 1989; Lairson and McGuire 1988; and Philbin and Altman, 1990). Case management differs according to need and socioeconomic resources. Since persons with AIDS are relatively young and insured through private insurance or Medicaid, hospice care may be free of the "six-month limit" that deters hospice use for persons with AIDS. Satisfaction of persons with AIDS with MCOs is comparable to their satisfaction with traditional insurers, except that MCO enrollees are less satisfied with their choice of clinicians and more satisfied with the cost of their insurance (Katz et al., 1997).

Alzheimer's disease, like AIDS, is an expensive, indolent, progressive disease. Its health care costs are about $90 billion. The most notable difference in health care financing between them is that Medicare is the major insurer for persons with dementia. Enrollees may switch back and forth between Medicare's fee-for-service and managed care option. Though 10% of Medicare beneficiaries are probably afflicted with Alzheimer's disease, MCOs are not a major insurer because a relatively small number of Medicare enrollees are in managed care and because MCOs rarely cover nursing home care. It is not known whether, or to what degree, persons with Alzheimer's disease self-select, or are steered to, the managed-care or fee-for-service arms of Medicare. It will probably not be cost-effective for MCOs to use new genetic tests for Alzheimer's disease for health insurance discrimination (Miles, 1998).

Alzheimer's disease, like AIDS, would be a likely choice for multidisciplinary case management if it were not for the fact that many community-based services are not well covered by Medicare. It is not likely that Medicare MCOs would pay for these services unless there were demonstrated cost-savings to the MCO in the form of less use of high cost services. Hospice is uncommonly used for demented persons because of incorrect fears that reimbursement to the program is at risk because the longevity of a person with dementia is unpredictable (Volicer et al., 1993; Scheetz, 1995; Hanrahan and Luchins, 1995, p. 1175; Hanrahan and Luchins, 1995, p. 47; Hanrahan and Luchins, 1995, p. 56). A large majority of professional and family caregivers of persons with dementia believe that hospice care is proper for endstage dementia (Luchins and Hanrahan, 1993). Successful hospice programs for dementia are financially viable, even for for-profit hospices (Volicer et al., 1986).

Case management for irreversible, indolent, progressive diseases poses the most challenging test of the health care, insurance regulation, and welfare systems. The variety of case management models for Alzheimer's disease and AIDS suggests that there is no consensus on the best way to handle these illnesses nor on core services that should be universally available. It is not clear whether an MCO should perform a broad biopsychosocial case management or whether it should be a member in a larger network of social programs and entitlements. This kind of illness imposes huge burdens on the loving caregivers of a person with this kind of illness (e.g., loss of wealth, income, housing, educational and health care opportunities for others) (Covinsky et al., 1994). These burdens shift costs from insurers or employers to lay caregivers and run counter to the public interests of maintaining healthy and productive family members.

A. Subacute Diseases: Cancer

Subacute, terminal diseases, like many untreatable and disseminated cancers, include persons who are recognized as dying for several months. There is little literature on how MCOs treat this pattern of dying. There is a substantial need to better identify people who have limited life expectancies in conditions like advanced heart failure or emphysema.

People needing subacute end-of-life care are vulnerable to becoming uninsured. Younger people who become debilitated and impoverished by costly out of pocket expenses or the loss of a job can be unable to pay insurance premiums. Insurance for older MCO Medicare members is more stable though the ability to afford Medicare supplemental policies to pay for community-based services or drugs decreases as resources are depleted by the extra costs of being ill. MCOs' Medicare members with cancer are not especially likely to disenroll and go to traditional Medicare where their providers are reimbursed on a fee-for-service basis (Riley et al., 1996). A recent study of Medicare found that persons with complex illness were being steered to fee-for service dying and persons with less expensive end-of-life needs were being steered to the capitated arm of Medicare (Morgan, 1997).

Hospices are responding to MCO market power (Mahoney, 1997). Some are vertically integrating: MCOs contract with hospices and in some cases provide or pay for most patients in their preferred hospices. Some compete for MCO referrals by taking less than the Medicare reimbursement and some MCOs or hospices reduce the hospice benefits for patients who are not on Medicare (Beresford, 1997). Such practices may adversely affect access to or the quality of hospice care. There are reports of MCOs dumping patients to hospices that the MCO does not fund, thereby shifting the costs of health care for that patient to out-of-pocket, or to public payers, or to voluntary services (Randal, 1996). Some hospices are joining into "horizontal" networks to collectively bargain with MCOs on rates and services (Beresford, 1995). There are few rigorous studies of the quality of subacute end-of-life care. In Great Britain, case management of terminally ill cancer patients produced small favorable changes in the quality of care (Addington-Hall et al., 1992).

B. Acute Catastrophic Dying

It is not known how many people die quickly after being briefly treated for a catastrophic injury or illness. Such persons often receive intense evaluation or treatment. Suicide, trauma, or firearms are collectively more frequent in the younger adults enrolled in MCOs. Fatal strokes or myocardial infarctions are more common in elderly adults. A study of California Medicare patients who had hospital care for the 15 most common causes of death, found that 5% of deaths occurred in patients who lived less than 100 days and had hospital expenses of more that $25000 (>90th percentile) (Cher and Henert, 1997).

There is concern about MCO cost-containment practices that affect treatment at the time of the catastrophe. Trauma centers are costly to operate and draw costly clients who are relatively more likely to need uncompensated care. MCOs have closed some trauma centers or emergency rooms but it is not clear how this has affected the provision of catastrophic end-of life care. Case reports describe how the perception that an MCO must be called before "911" has delayed emergency care and possibly caused death (Dickinson and Verdile, 1996). Legal reforms to assure that reasonable lay persons' perception of a medical emergency are sufficient to secure paid access to emergency care are being enacted by some states and by Congress. After adjusting for differences between the health of managed care and non-managed care populations, the treatment, outcomes and use of intensive care and "Level I" trauma care is not affected by insurance status (Angus et al., 1996; Waldrep et al., 1994; Pearson et al., 1994). In California, potentially ineffective care (very high cost care with short survival) is three-fourths as frequent among patients who are in managed Medicare as compared to fee-for-service Medicare. Some MCOs transfer patients in the middle of trauma or intensive care (Campbell et al., 1995). It is not clear whether such transfers improve treatment and physician–patient–family communication by returning a patient and family to a familiar hospital or harm treatment by removing them from established clinical relationships. Studies of the effects of case-managing intensive care at the end of life to improve the communication of advance directives or prognoses, their incorporation into treatment plans, the quality of pain control, or reduce costs have not found a major effect (SUPPORT Investigators, 1995; Miles et al., 1996).

4. THE COST-BENEFITS OF MANAGED END-OF-LIFE CARE

Market forces affect MCO end-of-life care. Mature managed care markets have decreased the oversupply of hospital beds. Those which also have a relatively high supply of physicians and competing large hospitals have more hospices (Chirikos and White, 1987). Markets with a high supply of hospitals provide more hospital-based end-of-life care (Pritchard, 1998). It is not clear whether hospices are created to contain costs, compete for market share, or simply compensate for a lack of hospital beds for end-of-life care. A study asking a small sample of Medicare enrollees to select potential benefits for Medicare coverage chose hospital and outpatient care, drugs, and preventive services. Hospice care was never a first choice and only 4% ranked it in their top three choices (Danis et al., 1997). Low consumer demand for end-of-life programs decreases the likelihood that consumer demand will be a powerful force on MCOs for improving their palliative care services.

The cost-benefits of managing end-of-life care are unclear. Most MCOs cover hospital care more adequately than nursing home or home care. Studies that only look at the cost of hospital care miss the important cost shifting that occurs when persons are transferred to public payers or to out-of-pocket spending for home care, hospice, or nursing homes. There is ample room for this cost-shifting: Medicare pays less than half of the last year of life expenditures for its enrollees (Institute of Medicine, 1997).

The heterogeneity of patients and programs makes it difficult to draw conclusions about cost savings from case managing chronic indolent diseases. For example, some MCOs assign the financial risk and the care of persons with AIDS to separate case-manager-providers (Knowlton, 1995); others keep these patients in the larger plan. A retrospective study found that case-managed persons with AIDS lived longer after diagnosis (533 days vs. 321 days) than non-case-managed persons and that case-managed care cost less ($11,143 vs. $20,523). Unfortunately, it compared case-managed private hospitals with non-case-managed public hospitals so that major socioeconomic differences between the groups, (despite controlling for race, alcohol use, IV drug abuse, and treatment with zidovudine) may have affected results (Sowell et al., 1992). Another study found that a public hospitals' AIDS patients had more needs for housing, nursing home, mental health and drug abuse treatment, than persons in community-based case management organizations though the latter had more difficulty obtaining home care, housekeeping and entitlements (Piette et al., 1990). MCOs have anecdotally reported savings from AIDS case-management ranging from $8000 to $56,000 over eighteen months (Kenkel, 1988) though Missouri found no diversion from hospital care (Twyman and Libbus, 1994).

The savings from managing indolent progressive end-of-life care in the elderly are also inconclusive. Irrespective of managed care, there is a trend to decreasing the role of the hospital in end-of-life care (McMillan et al., 1990). This trend is slightly accelerated for managed care Medicare patients (Gaumer and Stavins, 1992; Sager et al., 1989). A study of frail elderly with a 23% annual mortality found no cost savings for managed, compared to fee-for-service care, but the MCO spent 40% less on home care; Experton et al., 1996). A study of palliative long term care units for persons with dementia found greater restriction of life-sustaining treatments, greater comfort, shorter survival, and less resource use for patients with less advanced dementia (Volicer et al., 1994). Promoting long-term physician–patient relationships decreases the end-of-life costs for the frail elderly (Weiss and Blustein, 1996). Persons with Alzheimer's disease or late-stage AIDS impoverish themselves with out-of-pocket health care expenses and then often become dependent on public insurance, rather than private insurance (Snow, 1996; Westmoreland, 1995; Anonymous, 1996).

The cost effectiveness of managing the subacute pattern of care of dying with hospices is favorable, for now (Kidder, 1992; Emmanuel, 1996). A British study found savings from case management of terminal cancer care (Rafferty et al., 1996). It is unclear how much of this advantage is due to the hospice level of care, the possibly decreasing voluntary contributions of hospice volunteers, or differences in patients selecting this kind of care. Hospice savings are greater for programs that divert persons from hospital and nursing home care to short pre-death hospice stays. With longer hospice stays, hospice seems to be an expanded community-care benefit set and its cost advantage decreases. The cost advantage of hospice care could lessen with wider use of technologies like infusion pumps for analgesia.

Several studies have found little cost savings effect of high level acute care case management by providing diagnostic information, nurse facilitation of physician–patient–family communication, and/or advance treatment planning (SUPPORT Investigators, 1995). These studies are difficult to interpret (Emmanuel, 1996). Advance directives or orders to forgo high-technology care that are executed close to the time of death do not decrease end-of-life health care costs. Patients who have used such documents early in care to avoid hospital or intensive care unit admission are not "seen" in many such studies.

The debate over cost containment and the limiting of "futile," emerging, unvalidated, complementary, or even beneficial but very costly treatments that a patient desires is often discussed in MCOs (Tilford and Fiser, 1996; Jecker and Schneiderman, 1992; Bayer et al., 1983). Most of the "high cost of dying" of indolent progressive diseases arises from the cost of palliative or long-term care and not hospital treatment (Scitovsky, 1988). For persons with the subacute course of dying, a greater percentage of costs is spent on treatment in hospitals. Perhaps the relatively shorter time between a state of well-being and grave illness sets the stage for a preference for very aggressive attempts to prolong life for subacute illnesses until very shortly before death. Indolent diseases may give patients and families who are supported by counseling a greater acceptance of the terminal outcome and a greater likelihood of treatment that is more exclusively focused on palliative goals (Christakis and Escarce, 1996). This debate will test and shape the emerging structure of end-of-life care by MCOs because these life-and-death issues presented in the form of patient or family drive advocacy for unproved and costly rescue therapies will be heard in the context of public mistrust of patient advocacy in the new cost-conscious health care system.

5. CONCLUSION

It is premature to conclude how the tradeoffs between the potential benefits and dangers of managed health care are going to play out. For now, the answer is: "it depends" (Miller and Luft, 1997). It depends on which MCO, which employer, and which benefits are in the insurance contract. It depends on how responsibility for indigent or institutionalized dying persons, especially persons with indolent progressive disease, are transferred from private and federal insurers to strapped state Medicaid budgets. If Medicaid budgets are inadequate and employers use managed care to underinsure their employees (General Accounting Office, 1997), MCOs will appear responsible for the effects of the political decision to underfinance health care. It depends on how MCOs are held accountable for the quality of end-of-life care, including fair insurance practices, risk adjusting to pay for high-cost patients, implementing quality assurance programs, requiring public reporting of outcomes, enabling government and consumers to act on those outcomes, and health plans' responses to these pressures. This accountability will depend on the development of clear, usable ways to define, measure, and report quality.

Using paradigmatic terminal illnesses can facilitate reform by simplifying the diversity of end-of-life health care. There are other ways to simplify this complex problem as well. Eighty percent of deaths result from ten causes (heart disease, cancer, stroke, emphysema, accidents, pneumonia, diabetes, AIDS, suicide, and chronic liver disease). Targeting these conditions would improve end-of-life care for all persons. However, people die in various ways from the same "cause" of death. "Heart disease" causes a third of deaths but includes young persons resuscitated from a cardiac arrest who die days later of anoxic brain damage, persons dying of indolent heart failure, and profoundly demented persons who receive palliative care for a heart attack. (Dementia is listed as a "cause" of a misleadingly low 1% of deaths.) Alternatively, end-of-life care could be classified into "ideal" trajectories of dying: acute, subacute, and chronic courses. Our approach, using readily recognizable, common diseases to represent paradigmatic courses of dying need not be refined by research into such "ideal forms." More importantly, though clinicians provide particular treatments, MCOs provide sets of therapies or institutions. An MCO that demonstrated its success in meeting the needs for persons with our paradigmatic courses would be able to meet needs for many other people as well.

End-of-life health care is both a universal health care need and a neglected one. For birth, we expect integrated maternal screening; prenatal care; informed choices for midwives versus physician care, home and hospital births; birthing classes, childbirth, post-natal care of the mother and child and public health surveillance and action for bad outcomes. By contrast, we do not systematically identify persons at high risk of dying, educate them about the choices they face, connect the care of chronic disease with its terminal phase, or treat endemic bad outcomes (such as poor pain control) as a public health problem. The reform of managed end-of-life care will not occur as MCOs tinker with "treatments" but depends on how they coordinate and improve complex systems for multi-institutional and multi-provider health care. The intriguing similarity between models for caring for persons with AIDS and for frail or demented elderly hint at the contours of an integrated managed care delivery system capable of caring for dying people of all ages with diverse needs (Benjamin, 1988).

University of Minnesota
Minneapolis, Minnesota

NOTES

[1] This paper is supported by The Project on Death in America Faculty Scholars Program of the Soros Foundation (SHM) and the Robert Wood Johnson Foundation's National Task Force on End of Life Care in Managed Care which is based at the Center for Applied Ethics and Professional Practice, Education Development Center of which Mildred Solomon is the principal investigator.

[2] Grateful acknowledgement to Joanne Lynn and to Mildred Solomon for her comments on this manuscript. Thanks to Kara Parker, Bob Koepp, and Tim McIndoo for assistance with manuscript preparation.

REFERENCES

Addington-Hall, J.M. et al.: 1992, 'Randomized controlled trial of effects of coordinating care for terminally ill cancer patients', *British Medical Journal* 305, 1317–1322.

Angus, D.C. et al.: 1996, 'The effect of managed care on ICU length of stay: implications for Medicare', *The Journal of the American Medical Association* 276, 1075–1082.

Anonymous: 1996, 'A question of care: HMO officials and AIDS activists are divided over the quality of AIDS care', *Modern Healthcare* 26, 122, 124, 126–129.

Barnes, D.E. et al.: 1996, 'Industry-funded research and conflict of interest: an analysis of research sponsored by the tobacco industry through the Center for Indoor Air Research', *Journal of Health Politics* 21, 515–542.

Bayer, R. et al.: 1983, 'The care of the terminally ill: morality and economics', *New England Journal of Medicine* 309, 1490–1494.

Beresford, L.: 1997, 'The future of hospice in a reformed American health care system: What are the real questions?', *Hospice Journal* 13, 85–91.

Beresford, L.: 1995, 'Idealistic hospice industry confronts managed care', *Medicine & Health* 49, 1–4.

Brenner, P.R.: 1997, 'Issue of access in a diverse society', *Hospice Journal* 12, 9–16.

Campbell, A.R. et al.: 1995, 'Trauma centers in a managed care environment', *Journal of Trauma* 39, 246–251.

Cassel, C.K.: 1996, 'Overview on attitudes of physicians toward caring for the dying patient', in American Board of Internal Medicine, *Caring for the Dying: Identification and Promotion of Physician Competency*, American Board of Internal Medicine, Phil., 3–8.

Cher, D.J. et al.: 1997, 'Method of Medicare reimbursement and rate of potentially ineffective care of critically ill patients', *The Journal of the American Medical Association* 278, 1001–1007.

Chirikos, T.N. et al.: 1987, 'Competition in health care markets and the development of alternative forms of service delivery', *Health Politics* 8, 325–338.

Christakis, N.A. et al.: 1996, 'Survival of Medicare patients after enrollment in hospice programs', *New England Journal of Medicine* 335, 172–178.

Covinsky, K.E. et al.: 1994, 'The impact of serious illness on patients' families', *The Journal of the American Medical Association* 272, 1839–1844.

Daniels, N.: 1990, 'Insurability and the HIV epidemic: ethical issues in underwriting', *Milbank Quaterly* 68, 497–525.

Danis, M. et al.: 1997, 'Older Medicare enrollees' choices for insured services', *Journal of the American Geriatric Society* 45, 688–694.

Danis, M. et al.: 1991, 'A prospective study of advance directives for life-sustaining care', *New England Journal of Medicine* 324, 882–888.

Dickinson, E. et al.: 1996, 'Managed care organizations: a link in the chain of survival?', *Annals of Emergency Medicine* 28, 719–721.

Donaldson, M.S.: 1996, 'Measuring quality of care at end-of-life'. Prepared for Robert Wood Johnson Working Conference, copy on file with author.

Dossetor, J. et al.: 1994, 'Ethics of palliative care in the context of limited resources: an essay on the need for attitudinal change', *Journal of Palliative Care* 10, 39–42.

Emanuel, E.J.: 1992, 'Cost savings at the end-of-life: what do the data show?', *The Journal of the American Medical Association* 275, 1907–1914.

Emanuel, E.J. et al.: 1994, 'The economics of dying: the illusion of cost savings at the end-of-life', The *New England Journal of Medicine* 330, 540–544.

Employment Retirement Income Security Act, 29USC 1001–1461 (1974).

Experton, B. et al.: 1996, 'A comparison by payor/providor type of the cost of dying among frail older adults', *Journal of the American Geriatric Society* 44, 1098-1107.

Fade, A. et al.: 1995, 'Managed care and end-of-life decisions', *Trends in Health Care, Law & Ethics* 10, 97–100.

Frank, R. G. et al.: 1997, 'The politics and economics of mental health "parity" laws', *Health Affairs* 16, 108–119.

Gaumer, G.L. et al.: 1992, 'Medicare use in the last ninety days of life', *Health Services Resource* 25, 725–742.

General Accounting Office: 1997, 'Family Health Insurance', GAO/HEHS-97-35. U.S. Government Printing Office, Washington, DC.

Gostin, L.O. et al.: 1993, 'Privacy and security of personal information in a new health care system', *The Journal of the American Medical Association* 270, 2487–2493.

Haas, J.S. et al.: 1993, 'Discussion of preferences for life-sustaining care by persons with AIDS: predictors of failure in patient-physician communication', *Archives of Internal Medicine* 153, 1241–1248.

Hanrahan, P. et al.: 1995, 'Access to hospice care', *Journal of the American Geriatric Society* 43, 1175–1176.

Hanrahan, P. et al.: 1995, 'Access to hospice programs in end-stage dementia: a national survey of hospice programs', *Journal of the American Geriatric Society* 43, 56–59.

Hanrahan, P. et al.: 1995, 'Feasible criteria for enrolling end-stage dementia patients in home hospice care', *Hospice Journal* 10, 47–54.

Health Insurance Portability and Accountability Act, P.L. 104-191, H.R. 3103.

Hillman, A.L.: 1995, 'The impact of physician financial incentives on high-risk populations in managed care', *Journal of Acquired Immune Deficiency Syndrome and Human Retrovirology* 8, 23–30.

Institute of Medicine: 1997, *Approaching Death*, National Academy Press, Washington, D.C.

Japsen, B.: 1994, 'AIDS-care plan to reduce costs ... Midway Hospital Medical Center, Country Villa Service Corp.', *Modern Healthcare* 24, 13.

Jecker, N. et al.: 1992, 'Futility and rationing', *American Journal of Medicine*, 189–196.

Katz, M.H. et al.: 1997, 'Insurance type and satisfaction with medical care among HIV-infected men', *Journal of Acquired Immune Deficiency Syndrome and Human Retrovirology* 14, 35–43.

Kaveny, M.C.: 1998, 'Managed care, assisted suicide, and vulnerable poplulations', *Notre Dame Law Review* 73, 1275–1310.

Kenkel, P.J.: 1988, 'Health insurers turning to managed care to control growing cost of AIDS care', *Modern Healthcare* 18, 38–40.

Kidder, D.: 1992, 'The effects of hospice coverage on Medicare expenditures', *Health Services Resource* 27, 195–217.

Knowlton, D.L.: 1995, 'HIV care: a capitated alternative', *Journal of Acquired Immune Deficiency Syndrome & Human Retrovirology* 8, 74–79.

Lairson, P.D. et al.: 1988, 'Integration proves key in provider response to AIDS', *Business and Health* 5, 18–19.

Lamphere, J.A. et al.: 1997, 'The surge in Medicare managed care: an update', *Health Affairs* 16, 127–133.

Luchins, D.J. et al.: 1993, 'What is appropriate health care for end-stage dementia?', *Journal of the American Geriatric Society* 41, 25–30.

Lynn, J.: 1997, 'An 88-year-old woman facing the end-of-life', *The Journal of the American Medical Association* 277, 1633–1639.

Mahoney, J.J.: 1997, 'Hospice and managed care', *Hospice Journal* 12, 81–84.

McMillan, A. et al.: 1990, 'Trends and patterns in place of death for Medicare enrollees', *Health Care Finance Review* 12, 11–17.

Mechanic, D. et al.: 1996, 'The impact of managed care on patients' trust in medical care and their physicians', *The Journal of the American Medical Association* 275, 1693–1697.

Miles, S.H. et al.: 1996, 'Advance end-of-life treatment planning: a research review', *Archives of Internal Medicine* 156, 1–6.

Miles, S.H. et al.: 1995, 'End-of-life treatment in managed care: the potential and the peril', *West Journal of Medicine* 163, 302–305.

Miles, S.H.: 1998, 'Managed care and the genetic testing with Alzheimer's disease', in S. Post (ed.), Genetic Testing for Alzheimer's disease: Clinical and Ethical Issues, Johns Hopkins University Press, Baltimore.

Miller, R.H. et al.: 1997, 'Does managed care lead to better or worse quality of care?', *Health Affairs* 16, 7–25.

Morgan, R.O., Virnig, B.A., DeVito, C.A. and Persily, N.A.: 1997, 'The Medicare–HMO revolving door – the healthy go in and the sick go out', *New England Journal of Medicine*, 337, 169–175.

Morrison, R.S. and Meir, D.E.: 1995, 'Managed care at the end-of-life', *Trends in Health Care, Law & Ethics* 10, 91–96.

Padgug, R.A.: 1995, 'AIDS, risk adjustment, and health care financing in New York state', *Journal of Acquired Immune Deficiency Syndromes and Human Retrovirology* 8, 53–66.

Pawling-Kaplan, M. et al.: 1989, 'Hospice care for minorities: an analysis of a hospital-based inner city palliative care service', *American Journal of Hospice Care* 6, 13–21.

Pearson, S.D. et al.: 1994, 'The impact of membership in a health maintenance organization on hospital admission rates for acute chest pain', *Health Services Resource* 29, 59–74.

Philbin, P. et al.: 1990, 'HIV/AIDS home care: an HMO experience', *Caring* 9, 42–45.

Piette, J. et al.: 1990, 'A comparison of hospital and community case management programs for persons with AIDS', *Medical Care* 28, 746–755.

Pritchard, R.S. et al.: 1998, 'Influence of patient preferences, and local health system characteristics on the place of death', *Journal of the American Geriatrics Society* 46(10), 1242–50.

Rafferty, J.P. et al.: 1996, 'A randomized controlled trial of the cost-effectiveness of a district coordinating service for terminally ill cancer patients', *Palliative Medicine* 10, 151–161.

Randal, J.: 1996, 'Hospice services feel the pinch of managed care', *Journal of the National Cancer Institute* 88, 860–862.

Rennie, D.: 1997, 'Thyroid storm', *The Journal of the American Medical Association* 277, 1242–1243.

Riley, G. et al.: 1996, 'Disenrollment of Medicare cancer patients from health maintenance organizations', *Medical Care* 34, 826–836.

Riley, G. et al.: 1991, 'Enrollee health status under Medicare risk contracts: and analysis of mortality rates', *Health Services Resource* 6, 137–163.

Riley, G. et al.: 1987, 'The use and costs of Medicare services by cause of death', *Inquiry* 24, 233–244.

Rowland, D. et al.: 1996, 'Medicaid: moving to managed care', *Health Affairs* 15, 150–152.

Rubin, S.M. et al.: 1994, 'Increasing the completion of the durable power of attorney for health care – a randomized controlled trial', *The Journal of the American Medical Association* 271, 209–212.

Ryndes, T.: 1989, 'The coalition model of case management for care of HIV-infected persons', *Quality Review Bulletin* 15, 4–8.

Sachs, G.A et al.: 1991, 'Limiting resuscitation: emerging policy in the emergency medical system', *Annals of Internal Medicine* 114, 151–154.

Sager, M.A. et al.: 1989, 'Changes in the location of death after passage of Medicare's prospective payment systems', *New England Journal of Medicine* 320, 433–439.

Scheetz, A. et al.: 1995, 'Access to hospice care', *Journal of the American Geriatric Society* 43, 1174.

Scitovsky, A.A. et al.: 1990, 'Effects of the use of AZT on the medical care costs of persons with AIDS in the first 12 months', *Journal of Acquired Immune Deficiency Syndrome* 3, 904–912.

Scitovsky, A.A.: 1994, 'The high cost of dying revisited', *Milbank Quarterly* 72, 561–591.

Scitovsky, A.A.: 1988, 'Medical care in the last twelve months of life: the relation between age, functional status, and medical care expenditures', *Milbank Quarterly* 66, 640–660.

Shimm, D. et al: 1991, 'Conflict of interest and informed consent in industry-sponsored clinical trials', *Journal of Legal Medicine* 12, 477–513.

Snow, C.: 1996, 'Medicare HMOs develop plan for future of Alzheimer's programming', *Modern Healthcare* 26, 66–68, 70.

Sonsel, G.E.: 1989, 'Case management in a community-based AIDS agency', *Quality Review Bulletin* 15, 31–36.

Sowell, R.L.: 1995, 'Community-based HIV case management: challenges and opportunities', *Journal of the Association of Nurses in AIDS Care* 6, 33–40.

Sowell, R.L. et al.: 1992, 'Impact of case management on hospital charges of PWAs in Georgia', *Journal of the Association Nurses in AIDS Care* 3, 24–31.

Sowell, R.L. et al.: 1995, 'Integrated case management: the AIDS Atlanta Model', *Journal of Case Management* 4, 15–21.

Sowell, R.L. et al.: 1994, 'An integrated case management model: developing standards, evaluation, and outcome criteria', *Nurses Administrative Quarterly* 18, 53–64.

Sulmasy, D.P.: 1995, 'Managed care and managed death', *Archives of Internal Medicine* 155, 133–136.

SUPPORT Investigators: 1995, 'A controlled trial to improve care for seriously ill hospitalized patients: the study to understand prognoses and prefences for outcomes and risks of treatments', *The Journal of the American Medical Association* 274, 1591–1598.

Taravella, S.: 1988, 'Kaiser starts AIDS prevention program', *Modern Healthcare* 26, 27–28.

Tilford, J.M. et al.: 1996, 'Futile care in the pediatric intensive care unit: ethical and economic considerations', *Journal of Pediatrics* 128, 725–727.

Twyman, D.M. et al.: 1994, 'Case-management of AIDS clients as a predictor of total inpatient hospital days', *Public Health Nursing* 11, 1406–1411.

Volicer, B.J. et al.: 1993, 'Predicting short-term survival for patients with advanced Alzheimer's disease', *Journal of the American Geriatric Society* 41, 535–540.

Volicer, L. et al.: 1986, 'Hospice approach to the treatment of patients with advanced dementia of Alzheimer's type', *The Journal of the American Medical Association* 256, 2210–2213.

Volicer, L. et al.: 1994, 'Impact of special care unit for patients with advanced Alzheimer's disease on patients' discomfort and costs', *Journal of the American Geriatric Society* 42, 597–603.

Waldrep, D.J. et al.: 1994, 'Future shock: trauma in the managed care era', *American Surgeon* 60, 892–894.

Weiss, L.J. et al.: 1996, 'Faithful patients: the effect of long term physician patient relationships on the costs and use of health care by older Americans', *American Journal of Public Health* 86, 1742–1747.

Wenger, N.S. et al.: 1996, 'Using ethics-focused standardized performance measures to improve end-of-life care in managed care settings', prepared for Robert Wood Johnson Working Conference, copy on file with author.

Westmoreland, T.M.: 1995, 'AIDS and politics: death and taxes', *Bull NY Academy of Medicine* 72, 273–282.

Wolf, S.M.: 1997, 'Physician-assisted suicide in the context of managed care', *Duquesne Law Review* 35, 455–479.

Yox, S.B.: 1990, 'How has your HMO responded to AIDS?', *HMO Practice* 4, 122–123.

PART IV

VISIONS OF THE FUTURE FOR
PHYSICIAN-ASSISTED SUICIDE

KENNETH A. DE VILLE

PHYSICIAN-ASSISTED SUICIDE AND THE STATES: SHORT, MEDIUM AND LONG TERM

In *Washington et al. v. Glucksberg et al.* and *Vacco, Attorney General of New York et al. v. Quill et al.*, the United States (U.S.) Supreme Court was asked to determine whether a state's criminal prohibition of assisted suicide violated the Fourteenth Amendment of the U.S. Constitution. The court held that it did not (*Glucksberg*, 1997; *Vacco*, 1997). Simply stated, the court's June 1997 decisions in these two cases mean that the physician-assisted suicide (PAS) debate will move to state legislatures, to the realm of moral and social debate and to the arena of criminal and civil law. It is now within the power of voters and state legislatures to grant citizens legal access to physician-assisted suicide. Whether they will do so though, and how assisted suicide will actually evolve in practice will depend on an interlocking complex of social, legal and professional factors. Both the law as written and the law as practiced are influenced by the endemic social, legal and medical professional contexts in which the law is applied.

This essay will explore the likely impact on clinical practice of the Supreme Court's decision to let states resolve the physician-assisted suicide issue in their legislatures – in the short, medium and long term. History does not repeat itself, but the past *is* prologue and U.S. experiences with abortion, withholding life support, the law of self-defense, and capital punishment all provide some clue as to what society can expect regarding the physician-assisted suicide debate in the near and distant future. I will argue that the practice culture of medicine and the medical–legal environment of the U.S. will likely ensure that physician-assisted suicide proliferates only slowly, but that that same culture will allow it to ultimately emerge into an accepted, although still highly scrutinized option for sick and dying patients.

States can respond to *Glucksberg* and *Vacco* in one of three ways. First, some states will continue to prohibit explicitly the practice, just as the vast majority of states do now. Some current potential penalties for assisted suicide are quite severe. It is sometimes treated as the equivalent of murder or manslaughter (Mesiel, 1995, 478–487). Second, some states, after public and legislative debate, will allow physician-assisted suicide

Loretta M. Kopelman and Kenneth A. De Ville (eds.), Physician-Assisted Suicide, 171–186.
© 2001 *Kluwer Academic Publishers. Printed in Great Britain.*

under certain regulated conditions. Oregon's Death with Dignity Bill has now become law (Or. Rev. Stat., 1995). There have been dozens of bills introduced in other state legislatures that would have also legalized physician-assisted suicide under some limited conditions. A group of physicians, scholars and lawyers have drafted a comprehensive Model Assisted Suicide Statute (Baron et al., 1996). Thus, it is likely that Oregon will be joined by at least some states in legalizing regulated physician-assisted suicide. Finally, some state legislatures may pass no laws regarding physician-assisted suicide. Four states currently have no statutory laws regarding assisted suicide (Furrow et al., 1995). In these states, physician-assisted suicide *may* be prohibited as matter of common law but the legal status of the practice remains murky. As the national debate proceeds, some of these states will undoubtedly commit themselves definitively to either prohibition or legalization.

Thus, states must adopt one of three legal stances. They will: 1) clearly prohibit physician-assisted suicide; 2) allow physician-assisted suicide under limited circumstances; or 3) neither clearly prohibit nor allow physician-assisted suicide. The key point is that under each of these three scenarios, the law in action will be substantially different than the law as written (Tulskey et al., 1996). As a result, in the short to medium term, the legalization of physician-assisted suicide in several states will probably neither have the impact that advocates hope, nor the repercussions that critics fear. In the long term, however, neither the limitations on legal physician-assisted suicide nor the illegality of physician-assisted suicide in other states is likely to stop the gradual and marginally more public expansion of the practice. But this expansion of physician-assisted suicide does *not* necessarily suggest that physician-assisted suicide and euthanasia will become a common component of conventional medical practice.

In the short term, physician-assisted suicide will probably remain illegal in most jurisdictions. And in those states in which physician-assisted suicide remains clearly illegal, some physicians will continue to provide such aid to patients, just as some or many apparently do now. In one survey, for example, 828 responding physicians reported that they had treated 156 patients who had requested physician-assisted suicide. Thirty-eight of those patients received prescriptions from their physicians to aid their death, of which 21 died as a result. Fifty-eight patients in the study requested euthanasia, fourteen of whom died after receiving parenteral medication (Back et al., 1996; Choen et al., 1994). Another survey of 1,902 physicians in ten different specialty practice areas concluded that 3.3 percent of physicians surveyed had written at least one prescription to hasten a patient's death and 4.7 percent had administered at least one lethal injection (Laino, 1998).

Despite the illegality of assisted suicide in virtually all jurisdictions, if physicians are discovered providing such assistance in dying to patients, they probably will not be prosecuted. If they are prosecuted, they will likely not be convicted. Past experience with the prosecution of physicians for aid in dying should make that clear. Consider the legacy of failed cases of prosecution for assisted suicide and euthanasia. Similarly, a New York grand jury refused to indict Timothy Quill for assisted suicide even though he appeared to admit it in the pages of the *New England Journal of Medicine* (Quill and Cassell, 1992). Michigan failed to convict Jack Kevorkian, even though he flagrantly defied the law, even though the state enacted a statute specifically aimed at his activity, even though he is suspected in some cases of euthanasia and not physician-assisted suicide, and even though some of his clients have suffered from nothing more than chronic fatigue syndrome and asymptomatic multiple sclerosis (D'Oronzio, 1996; Morgan and Sutherland, 1996). Kevorkian admittedly participated in scores of suicides but it was not until he allowed a videotaped account of him actually administering a lethal injection on the network television show "60 Minutes" – i.e., engaging in euthanasia, not merely physician-assisted suicide – that Kevorkian was finally convicted of second degree murder (Johnson, 1999). Similarly, in September of 1997, a Florida jury refused to convict Dr. Ernesto Pinzon-Reyes of homicide. Pinzon-Reyes personally injected a terminal patient with a combination of valium, potassium chloride, and morphine. A nurse had warned the physician moments before that the injection would kill the patient and the family supported the prosecutor's attempts to convict the physician (Associate Press, September 9, 1997). The overall legal history of assisted suicide, mercy killing and euthanasia confirms that prosecutors and grand juries typically refuse to indict and juries refuse to convict if trial is reached, whether the perpetrator is a physician or a layperson (Glantz, 1987; Shaffer, 1986; Gostin, 1993). Leonard Glantz has found only twenty prosecutions for mercy killing and assisted suicide from 1939 through 1983. Only three resulted in convictions, and those involved non-physicians. Moreover, the rare convictions that are secured for euthanasia or mercy killing invariably result in trivial penalties. Few of these prosecutions for mercy killing involved physicians, and there have been no convictions of physicians for assisted suicide (Stone and Winslade, 1995).

There are a number of reasons why physician-assisted suicide prosecutions have proven consistently problematic. The first is so-called "jury nullification." A significant minority of public opinion, at least, favors physician-assisted suicide (Blendon et al., 1992). It would be difficult to empanel a jury on which there were not at least some members who are sympathetic to physician-assisted suicide and who might be willing to ignore the law or facts in order to benefit a physician-defendant. And, it only takes one juror to "hang" a jury. This mixed public attitude aggravates other problems endemic to the prosecution of physician-assisted suicide cases. Many or most of the physicians who participate in physician-assisted suicide or mercy killing are probably "attractive" or sympathetic defendants who appear to have acted for beneficent, patient-centered reasons. They may be friends of the family or the deceased and may appear to have little to gain from their actions. In many cases it may be difficult to demonstrate that the physician-defendant's actions meet the required elements of the criminal offense. For example, did the physician "intend" to end the life of the patient, or merely end his or her pain? Criminal law holds that individuals are presumed to intend the logical consequences of their actions, but juries may be unwilling to apply this doctrine with precision in cases where the patient was also suffering great pain. In addition, there are often causality and other evidentiary problems. When patients are very ill, as they frequently are in physician-assisted suicide cases, it is not always easy to prove what, in fact, caused the patient's death. For example, medical experts testified in the Pinzon-Reyes Florida homicide trial that the physician's injections probably did not cause death, and if they did it would be difficult to prove given the patient's near death condition and the fact that the body had been embalmed before examination (Associated Press, September 9, 1997). Similarly, a respiratory therapist in California recently confessed to killing nearly fifty patients. Even with a list of putative victims and a confession, officials have been unsure if they will be able to prosecute successfully the therapist. Decreased oxygen settings on ventilator dependent patients cannot be proven. Many drugs break-down quickly in the system and are virtually untraceable if the patient lives for even a short time after injection. And, Quill and Kevorkian aside, physicians seldom advertise lawbreaking. As a result, collecting conclusive evidence on the assisted suicide of an extremely elderly or terminal patient could be nearly impossible. Cyril Wecht, a leading figure in forensic pathology, has noted the intrinsic difficulty in determining the cause of death in severely ill patients. As Wecht observes: "Who in the hell knows when such people die, they could die any day anyway" (Fleeman, 1998). Finally, the prosecution of physician-assisted suicide and mercy killing cases may represent a double-edged political liability for the elected district attorney: 1) because much of the public supports physician aid in dying and would resent the prosecution of physician-assisted suicide cases (Furrow et al., 1995, p. 420); and 2) because those individuals opposed to physician-assisted suicide might hold the district attorney responsible for failing to convict and punish physicians who break the law. Thus, even in states where physician-assisted suicide is clearly illegal, it will continue to be difficult to charge and convict physicians who help their patients to die.

But the illegality of physician-assisted suicide is not irrelevant. Some physicians will still have to face prosecution, a profoundly unpleasant prospect. Even if they are ultimately acquitted, they will, as courtroom pundits note, "beat the rap but not the ride." Thus potential prosecution, even that which is likely to result in acquittal, will serve as a strong disincentive to widespread, open physician-assisted suicide in states where the practice is considered a criminal offense. Some physicians will be deterred from acting in *any* way that might be construed as assisted suicide; others will limit their clandestine participation to a very narrow range of cases.

In the few states where legislatures have not acted, and where the legal status of physician-assisted suicide is a matter of common law or unclear, the results will largely be the same. If prosecutors cannot sustain physician-assisted suicide convictions in jurisdictions where the practice is clearly illegal, then it will surely not be possible in jurisdictions where there is no explicit statutory law prohibiting it. Still, the illegal or uncertain legal status of physician-assisted suicide will discourage most physicians from acting, though many will continue to provide physician-assisted suicide undercover.

To date, only Oregon has legalized physician-assisted suicide, but, given significant public support for the practice, there are undoubtedly more states to come. A 1993 national survey revealed that 44% of those questioned were in favor of legalized physician-assisted suicide and 55% for euthanasia (Johnson, 1996, p. 25). A 1994 Harris poll found that 70% of the population favored assisted suicide including 90% of people with

AIDS (Batavia, 1997). In 1994, the electorate in Washington and California only narrowly defeated a proposal that would legalize not only physician-assisted suicide but also active euthanasia (Misbin, 1991).

All proposals to legalize physician-assisted suicide have included a series of statutorily defined safeguards that must be satisfied before a physician can provide a patient with the means to end his or her own life. In Oregon for example, among other requirements, the patient seeking aid in dying must be "terminal," "competent" and informed of all available alternatives to physician-assisted suicide. The patient must request assistance in dying orally and in writing and there is a mandatory 15 day waiting requirement between requests. The attending physician must consult with a second physician in order to secure written confirmation of the patient's competence and terminal condition. Oregon's physician-assisted suicide statute also has a variety of documentation requirements; and physician-assisted suicide records will be reviewed by state regulators annually (Or. Rev. Stat., 1995).

Opponents of physician-assisted suicide argue that numerous Oregon safeguards are ambiguous and will lead to abuses, or at least a likely expansion of the practice to a much broader class of cases (Johnson, 1996, p. 30). For example, the 1997 New York State Task Force on Life and the Law concluded that legalizing physician-assisted suicide "would pose serious and insurmountable risks of mistake and abuse that would greatly outweigh any benefit that might be achieved" (New York State Task Force, 1997, p. 1). As the Task Force's report notes:

> The clinical safeguards that have been proposed to prevent abuse and errors are unlikely to be realized in everyday medical practice. Moreover, the private nature of these decisions would undermine efforts to monitor physicians' behavior and prevent mistakes (New York State Task Force, 1997, p. 5).

Task force members argued that if physician-assisted suicide is accepted for one group – the terminal, competent patient – there is no principled basis or bright line test on which to deny other individuals access to physician-assisted suicide or even euthanasia.

These concerns (and fears like them) may be well founded. Many of the regulations *are* ambiguous, leaving considerable room for either differing interpretations or expansion of what is currently accepted practice (Capron, 1995). But ironically, the same ambiguity that conjures up visions of a slippery slope will likely keep many physicians from participating in physician-assisted suicide at all, at least in the short run. Some advocates of physician-assisted suicide, for example, are concerned that proposed physician-assisted suicide statutes, filled with bureaucratic safeguards, demand too much from terminal patients and their physicians and will thus thwart individuals who wish to take advantage of the statute. But that is not the only potential problem. Consider the requirement that the patient be "terminal." There is little agreement medically or legally as to what constitutes "terminal." State advance directive laws define the term in a variety of different ways: e.g., death will occur in a "relatively short period of time" or death is "imminent" (Marzen, 1994). A terminal condition, according to the Oregon statute, is one in which the patient will die of his or her underlying illness within six months. But even with this guidance, "terminal" remains a highly subjective and unverifiable predication about the future, especially if the patient takes advantage of physician-assisted suicide to end his or her life before the underlying illness runs its course. Potential complications abound. Does terminal mean with treatment, or without treatment? Clearly the other treatment decisions made by the patient and health care team will often have a major impact on life expectation. A patient might reasonably be considered terminal without the use of antibiotics, chemotherapy or dialysis, but not necessarily qualify as terminal if those modalities are employed. Most proposed physician-assisted suicide legislation provides no guidance on this issue. Even if a consensus is reached on what terminal means, physicians' ability to predict the likely time of death is notoriously poor (Evans and McCarthy, 1985).

Other terminology is similarly problematic. What does "competency" mean in the context of wishing to make an irrevocable decision about ending one's life? What does it mean legally? Medically? Physicians, psychiatrists and judges have rarely been asked to determine an individual's competency under these circumstances. Determinations of competency in right-to-refuse life-sustaining treatment situations may, of course, provide some analogical guidance, but even there the context is distinguishable (Youngner, 1998). Other proposed regulations generate similar ambiguities. The Model Physician-Assisted Suicide statute, for example, sanctions physician aid in dying if the patient is terminal or is a victim of "unbearable suffering." Unbearable suffering seems an even more subjective and vague guide than does the terminal standard. The evaluation of pain in other contexts has proven extraordinarily problematic, in the evaluation of disability payments for example

(Johnson, 1996, p. 28). Pain is perceived and borne by different individuals in different degrees. Adding to the puzzle, the Model Physician-Assisted Suicide statute appears to allow consideration of the highly idiosyncratic notion of mental and psychic suffering in determining whether physician-assisted suicide is justified. As the New York State Task Force on Life and the Law concluded, "neither pain nor suffering can be gauged objectively or subjectively to the kind of judgments needed to fashion a coherent public policy [on physician-assisted suicide]" (New York State Task Force, 1994, p. 132). Even simpler terms take on a new complexity in the context of physician-assisted suicide. Oregon requires that individuals who wish to take advantage of the statute be "residents" of the state. Although residency requirements vary from state to state, in many, residency merely requires the intent of the individual to establish a permanent domicile in the particular jurisdiction. Whether there is sufficient evidence of that "intent" becomes a matter of interpretation (Capron, 1995).

These interpretive ambiguities, and others, will make some physicians hesitant to provide physician-assisted suicide even in jurisdictions where the practice is legal because they will be uncertain that they have fulfilled all the legal requirements and because they fear liability, both criminal and civil. Indeed, opponents of euthanasia and physician-assisted suicide are advocating the use of civil, medical malpractice sanctions to discourage physicians from aiding their patients' suicides (Balch and O'Steen, 1997). Minnesota, Tennessee, North Dakota, and Virginia have already passed specific statutes allowing the recovery of civil damages from physicians engaging in physician-assisted suicide. However, no specific statute is required for an angry family member with standing (a child or parent) to file a suit claiming that physician-assisted suicide does not conform to the medical community's standard of care, and thus constitutes medical malpractice. The American Medical Association's Council on Ethical and Judicial Affairs has condemned the practice declaring that: "Physician-assisted suicide is fundamentally incompatible with the physician's role as healer, would be difficult or impossible to control, and would pose serious societal risks" (AMA, 1997). In its 1998 annual meeting, the American Society of Anesthesiologists declared its official opposition to assisted suicide "in favor of current treatments that reduce pain in terminally ill patients" (AMA, 1998). Families might also find powerful allies in state medical societies that oppose the practice. Although civil malpractice claims would not be strong (especially in jurisdictions where physician-assisted suicide is legal) and would face the same hurdles as criminal prosecutions for assisted suicide, the theoretical risk of civil suit will undoubtedly discourage some physicians from participating in the practice.

Physicians who act under physician-assisted suicide statutes are protected legally and probably run no risk of prosecution, even in close cases; nonetheless most physicians will likely be overcautious. Consider how physicians have responded to patient requests to withdraw life-sustaining treatment. Many have delayed legitimate patient and family requests for fear of litigation. Physicians are likely to be far more wary of physician-assisted suicide which is clearly on shakier ground legally and ethically than the right to refuse treatment. State medical societies may also blunt proliferation of the practice. Physicians who have participated in physician-assisted suicide and euthanasia have lost their licenses and their privilege to practice medicine (National Law Journal, 1998). Pinzon-Reyes, the physician exonerated by a Florida jury, was still fighting the state medical board to restore his license over two years after his acquittal for manslaughter. Although the potential loss of one's medical license would probably not discourage Jack Kevorkian, or physicians like him, it might deter other physicians who wish to maintain their more traditional medical practice and patient pool. Medical institutions, are typically wary of practices and behaviors that may subject them to litigation or public relations disasters. Such institutional circumspection will likely slow proliferation of open physician-assisted suicide further. Many institutions will not see it in their interest to be viewed as the physician-assisted suicide center of their city or region. This caution may be especially apparent at institutions that serve patient populations that are traditionally suspicious of the medical profession and institutionalized physician-assisted suicide. Thus, like abortion, legalized physician-assisted suicide may become marginalized in a few institutions limited access to the practice.

Some observers fear what they view as the unholy alliance of managed care and physician-assisted suicide (Sulmasy, 1995). While these fears should be taken seriously, managed care organizations (MCOs) and physician-assisted suicide may not be the natural and immediate allies that many believe. Even cost-conscious MCOs may embrace physician-assisted suicide only warily. While MCOs clearly have an interest in limiting the costs at the end of life, they are unlikely in the short term to aggravate their already tarnished public image by an enthusiastic embracing of physician-assisted suicide. Some segments of the public already believe that MCOs tend to place profits over patient interests. Savvy executives are unlikely to feed that sentiment further. Moreover, the cost savings associated with the acceptance of physician-assisted suicide may not be nearly as large as some observers speculate. A study by Ezekiel Emanuel and Peggy Battin concludes that assisted suicide, legalized nationally, would represent a cost savings equal to *at most* 0.07 percent of the total health care expenditures of the nation. As a result, they note, "Physician-assisted suicide is not likely to save substantial amounts of money in absolute or relative terms, either for particular institutions or for the nation as a whole (Emanuel and Battin, 1998). Thus, even rapacious health care institutions may only warily pursue physician-assisted suicide given the attendant potential public relations risks and probably only modest financial rewards.

Other factors, too, may make physicians hesitant to proceed with aid in dying even where physician-assisted suicide is legal and the legal technicalities have been relatively clearly satisfied. Medical teams may defer patients' requests for aid in dying where any member of the immediate family protests. This pattern has been true with organ donations, validly executed living wills, and oral requests to refuse treatment from competent patients. A combination of respect for family wishes and excessive litigation wariness have frequently slowed or blocked acceptance of a patient's clearly expressed wishes. In addition, there may be federal law considerations that slow implementation of legalized physician-assisted suicide. The Federal Controlled Substances Act, for example, requires that pharmaceuticals be prescribed for a "legitimate therapeutic purpose." It is, at this point, unclear if physician-assisted suicide is a "legitimate" medical purpose given that the drafters of the Federal Controlled Substances Act almost certainly did not have physician-assisted suicide in mind at the time of the enactment of the statute. Indeed, the U.S. Drug Enforcement Agency initially warned that Oregon physicians who prescribed drugs for assisted suicide could lose their federal right to prescribe (Associated Press, March 25, 1998). Justice Department officials have since indicated, however, that such interventions are unlikely. Federal and state funding limitations may also play a role in limiting the widespread use of physician-assisted suicide. The Assisted-Suicide Federal Funding Restrictions Act of 1996, for example, denied the use of any federal funds for physician-assisted suicide services. This bill failed as did the so-called "Lethal Drug Prevention Act of 1998" (Gianelli, 1998).

As importantly, new and additional safeguards are likely to be added to physician-assisted suicide as the political process proceeds and the public debate continues. On one hand, new safeguards may assuage the fears of those voters and health professionals who agree with physician-assisted suicide in principle, but fear abuses and mistakes. On the other hand, the more safeguards that are added, the more slowly physician-assisted suicide may proliferate. The mere presence of additional regulations will be more burdensome for clinicians. Moreover, each new qualification will carry its own ambiguity and generate additional uncertainty. More extensive and explicit reporting requirements could have a chilling effect on how openly the practice occurs. Each additional layer of required consultation could add a layer of legal fear, founded and unfounded. For example, some physician-assisted suicide proposals require psychiatric consultations to determine that the patient is competent and/or not suffering from clinical depression. Other observers have recommended a mandatory palliative care consultation, as well as a second medical opinion (Miller et al., 1996). Each of the professionals involved in certifying that the patient is a legal candidate for physician-assisted suicide, may question their role in the process, including its potential (albeit only hypothetical) legal danger. As a result, legal and regulated physician-assisted suicide will be complicated even further.

Thus in the short term, the effect of regulated and legalized physician-assisted suicide will be paradoxical. It will be impossible to define unambiguously a class of patients eligible for physician-assisted suicide (Coleman and Fleischman, 1996). This failure has very little to do with physician-assisted suicide and everything to do with what happens when regulatory law interacts with the medical practice culture. Regulatory law in general is alternatively too vague to be useful or too specific to provide definitive and wise guidance in real-life medical practice. I believe, however, that the ambiguity in physician-assisted suicide guidelines will cut *two* ways. It will probably slow utilization among many physicians. But at the same time, as opponents of physician-assisted suicide fear, it probably will mean that the practice sometimes extends beyond state guidelines, to the so-called slippery slope.

Unlike some analyses, these comments are not a claim that physician-assisted suicide is non-regulatable (Callahan and White, 1996), or that regulations are irrelevant. But medical professionals, the public, and

policy makers should be sensitive to the fact that there will inevitably be a
broad range of discretion and uncertainty involved in the application of
laws allowing *or* prohibiting the practice (or virtually any other practice
for that matter). Consider, as analogy, the dynamics of highway speed
limits. State imposed speed limits serve a regulatory function, but they do
not hold people necessarily to the posted limit in all conditions and in all
cases (Haber, 1996). Similarly, state legislation allowing, but regulating,
physician-assisted suicide will play an important role in limiting the
application and growth of the practice even if physician-assisted suicide
is not contained within the strict guidelines of the statute.

In the medium to long term, the practice of physician-assisted suicide
will evolve and expand by a slow accumulation of individual decisions
and greater open discussion of the practice. After all, some cases *will* fall
clearly under the guidelines and some physicians will dare to act. One
study, for example, reported that, if legal, 36 percent of the physicians
polled would provide physician-assisted suicide and 24 percent would
administer injections to hasten patients' deaths (Laino, 1998). When
physicians who aid their patients to die are not punished, and that
behavior is publicized, such actions will undoubtedly increase. Moreover,
as opponents of the practice fear, some physicians will exploit the
ambiguity in physician-assisted suicide statutes and gradually expand the
practice (Meisel, 1998, p. 820). This process, however, will likely occur
only slowly and take a matter of years, rather than a matter of months. It
is significant that the first publicly acknowledged assisted suicide under
the Oregon act did not occur until six months after the law took effect
(Associated Press, March 25, 1998). In its first year of operation, the use
of Oregon's assisted suicide statute led to only 15 deaths (Chin et al.,
1999). As several scholars have argued, decriminalization will not
necessarily make suicide and assisted suicide suddenly more acceptable
and less socially stigmatized. Decriminalization of suicide has not led to
widespread social acceptance and implicit encouragement of the practice
even over many years. In fact, in the years since decriminalization,
society has expended tremendous social resources in preventing suicides
(Stone and Winslade, 1995).

The practice is also likely to increase because I believe more states are
likely to enact physician-assisted suicide laws as time passes. Many states
are already considering such action. There is significant public support
for the practice and it will likely continue because I predict that abuses
either will not be spectacular and numerous, or will be hidden. In the

wake of *Glucksberg* and *Vacco*, measures legalizing physician-assisted suicide have been rejected in over 20 state legislatures (Verhovek, 1999). In the long run, however, I believe that the public and the profession will slowly come to tolerate its existence. I stress tolerate, because despite this toleration, I believe that physician-assisted suicide will remain a stigmatized event professionally and socially, much like abortion. (Admittedly though, the degree to which physician-assisted suicide is stigmatized in any particular instance may depend upon a variety of factors including the reasons for which it is pursued.) Physicians may be hesitant to participate not only as the result of legal fears but also in consideration of what such participation might mean for their practice. Will patients who oppose the practice avoid them out of fear or moral revulsion? Will a practitioner who is willing to provide the service suddenly become the physician in their locale to whom all patients requesting death are referred? As a result of these and other factors, most physicians will not offer physician-assisted suicide to their patients even if they may be willing to refer interested and eligible patients to physician-colleagues who will provide physician-assisted suicide. This professional hesitance will be aggravated by the fact that training for physician-assisted suicide euthanasia will probably *not* occur in medical schools – much in the way that abortion training is not offered in the majority of residency programs. And, as with abortion, protests by right-to-life groups will likely escalate stigmatizing the practice further.

CONCLUSION

In the long term, the slippery slope, in one sense, will become a reality. Physician-assisted suicide and maybe even euthanasia will be extended to non-terminal and incompetent patients in at least a narrowly defined range of circumstances. That is a prediction, not necessarily a celebration, a descriptive, not a normative conclusion. At the same time, however, we take death very seriously in this country, in the social, legal and medical environments. That is not likely to change even in the long-term. And, as a result, physician-assisted suicide and euthanasia are not likely to become a common component of conventional medical practice. In closing, consider two other areas of state-sanctioned death: capital punishment and self-defense. One, capital punishment, is highly regulated with mind-numbing specificity. In part as a result, it is relatively rarely used. In contrast, the use of deadly force in self-defense is legally justified only if "the force employed is reasonable in relation to the threat." But the exceptionally vague guideline that regulates self-defense has not led to widespread vigilantism and irate property owners shooting bicycle thieves. Likewise, in the long run, while I think physician-assisted suicide, and perhaps limited euthanasia will be ultimately legal in a significant number of jurisdictions, it will remain only tolerated by the medical profession and a significant portion of society.

Brody School of Medicine at East Carolina University
Greenville, North Carolina

REFERENCES

AMA Council on Ethical and Judicial Affairs: 1997, *Code of Medical Ethics, Current Opinions with Annotations*, Opinion 2.211.

American Medical Association: 1998, 'Anesthesiologists: no doctor-assisted suicide,' *American Medical News*, Nov. 23–Nov. 30, 1998, 41, 19.

Associated Press: Sept. 9, 1997, 'Controversy arises over cause of death,' http//www.sunsentinel.com/daily/5658.htm.

Associated Press: March 25, 1998, 'Oregon woman takes advantage of assisted suicide law,' Associated Press, http://www.cnn.com/US/9803/25/assisted.suicide.ap.

Back, A.L. et al.: 1996, 'Physician-assisted suicide and euthanasia in washington state: patient requests and physician responses', *The Journal of the American Medical Association* 275,12, 919–925.

Balch, B.J. and O'Steen, D.N.: 1997, 'Why we shouldn't legalize assisting suicide, part IV: the need for civil remedies to prevent assisting suicide,' National Right to Life Committee, http://www.nrlc.org/euthanasia/asisend4.html.

Baron, C.H. et al.: 1996, 'A model state act to authorize and regulate physician-assisted suicide,' *Harvard Journal of Legislation* 33, 1–34.

Batavia, A.I.: 1997, 'Disability and the physician-patient relationship,' *New England Journal of Medicine* 336, 23, 1671–1673.

Blendon, R.J., Szalay U.S., and Knox R.A.: 1992, 'Should physicians aid their patients in dying? the public perspective,' *The Journal of the American Medical Association* 267, 2658–2662.

Callahan, D. and White, M.: 1996, 'The legalization of physician-assisted suicide: creating a regulatory Potemkin Village,' *University of Richmond Law Review* 30, 1–83.

Capron, A.M.: January–February 1995, 'Sledding Oregon,' *Hastings Center Report*, 34–35.

Chin, A.E., Hedberg, K., Higgonson G.K., and Fleming, D.W.: 1999, 'Legalized physician-assisted suicide in Oregon – the first year's experience,' *New England Journal of Medicine* 340(7): 577–583.

Cohen, J.S., Fihn, S.D., Boyko E.J., Jonsen A.R., and Wood, R.W.: 1994, 'Attitudes toward assisted suicide and euthanasia among physicians in Washington State,' *New England Journal of Medicine* 331, 1240–1243.

Coleman, C.H. and Fleischman, A.R.: 1996, 'Guidelines for physician-assisted suicide: can challenge be met?' *Journal of Law Medicine & Ethics* 24, 217–224.

D'Oronzio, J.C.: 1996, 'Repelling on the slippery slope: negotiating public policy for physician-assisted death,' *Cambridge Quarterly of Health Care Ethics* 6, 113–117.

Emanuel E.J., Battin M.P.: 1998, 'What are the potential cost savings from legalizing physician-assisted suicide?' *New England Journal of Medicine* 339(3): 167–172.

Evans C., McCarthy M.: 1985, 'Prognostic uncertainty in terminal care: can the Karnofsky index help?' *Lancet* 1 (8439): 1204–1206.

Fleeman, M.: March 30 1998, 'Hospital killings tough to prove,' Associated Press, http://search.washington post.com/wp-srv/WAPA/19980330/V000132-03398-idx.html.

Furrow, B.R., Greaney, T.L., Johnson, S.H., Jost, T.S., and Schwartz, R.L.: 1995, *Health Law*, West Publishing Company, St. Paul, Minnesota, Volume 2, p. 420.

Gianelli, D.M.: 1998, 'Backdoor ban on suicide aid hits impasse,' *American Medical News*, 41(41): 8–9.

Glantz, L.H.: 1987, 'Withholding and withdrawing treatment: the role of the criminal law,' *Law, Medicine & Health Care* 15, 231–241.

Gostin, L.O.: 1993, 'Drawing a line between killing and letting die: the law, and law reform, on Medically Assisted Dying,' *Journal of Law Medicine and Ethics* 21, 1, 94–100.

Haber, J.G.: 1996, 'Should the physicians assist the reaper,' *Cambridge Quarterly of Health Care Ethics* 5, 44–49 at 48.

Johnson, D.: 1999, 'Kevorkian sentenced to 10 to 25 years in prison,' *New York Times*, April 14, 1999, p. A1.

Johnson, S.: 1996, 'Setting limits on death: A view from the United States,' *Cambridge Quarterly of Healthcare Ethics* 5, 24–32.

Laino, C.: 1998, 'Physician-assisted suicide still rare,' *MSNBC Health News*, <http://www.msnbc.com/news/160366.asp>, accessed July 16, 1998.

Marzen, T. J.: 1994, 'Out, out brief candle: constitutionally prescribed suicide for the terminally ill,' *Hastings Law Quarterly* 21, 799–826.

Meisel, A.: 1995, *The Right to Die Second Edition*, vol. 2, John Wiley & Sons, Inc, New York, pp. 478–487.

Meisel, A.: 1997, 'Physician-assisted suicide: a common law roadmap for state courts,' *Fordham Urban Law Journal*, 23, pp. 817–857.

Miller, F.G., Brody, H. and Quill, T.E.: 1996, 'Can physician-assisted suicide be regulated effectively?' *Journal of Law, Medicine & Ethics* 24, 225–232.

Misbin, RI.: 1991, 'Physician's aid in dying,' *New England Journal of Medicine* 325, 1307–1311.

Morgan, R. and Sutherland, D.D.: 1996, 'Last rights? confronting physician assisted suicide in law and society,' *Stetson Law Review* 26, no. 2, 481–528.

National Law Journal: 1998 'Suicide doctor expelled,' *National Law Journal*, March 30, 1998, A 12.

New York State Task Force on Life and the Law: 1997, *When Death is Sought: Assisted Suicide and Euthanasia in the Medical Context, Supplement to Report*, State Task Force on Life and the Law, New York, New York.

New York State Task Force on Life and the Law: 1994, *When Death is Sought: Assisted Suicide and Euthanasia in the Medical Context*, New York State Task Force on Life and the Law, New York.

Oregon Death with Dignity Act, *Or. Rev. Stat.* secs. 127.00 *et seq.* (1995).

Quill, T. and Cassel, C.: 1992, 'Care of the hopelessly ill: Proposed clinical criteria for physician-assisted suicide,' *New England Journal of Medicine* 327, 1380–1381.

Shaffer, C.D.: 1986, 'Criminal liability for assisting suicide,' *Columbia Law Review* 86, 348, 369–371.

Stone, T. H. and Winslade, W.J.: 1995, 'Physician-assisted suicide and euthanasia in the United States: legal and ethical observations,' *The Journal of Legal Medicine* 16, 481–507.

Sulmasy, D.P.: 1995, 'Managed care and managed death,' *Archives of Internal Medicine* 155, 133–136.

Tulsky, J.S., Alpers, A., and Lo, B.: 1996, 'A middle ground on physicians assisted suicide,' *Cambridge Quarterly of Health Care* 5, 33–43.

Vacco, Attorney General of New York et al. v. Quill et al., 117 S. Ct. 2293 (1997).

Verhovek, S.H.: 1999, 'Oregon reporting 15 deaths in 1998 under suicide law,' *New York Times*, Feb. 18, 1998, A1.

Washington, et al. v. Glucksberg, et al., 117 S. Ct. 2258 (1997).

Youngner S.L.: 1998, 'Why psychiatrists shouldn't be the gatekeepers for physician assisted suicide,' Paper Delivered at Spring Meeting of the Society for Health and Human Values, Greenville, N.C., March 13, 1998.

MARGARET P. BATTIN

SAFE, LEGAL, RARE? PHYSICIAN-ASSISTED SUICIDE
AND CULTURAL CHANGE IN THE FUTURE[1]

Cultural change is well recognized in the recent history of death and
dying. In the wake of Elizabeth Kübler-Ross's 1969 work *On Death and
Dying*, not only has it become socially acceptable to talk about death and
dying with someone who is terminally ill, but, as traditional religious and
legal strictures loosen, it is becoming possible for a person facing death to
consider what role he or she wants to play in the forthcoming death. The
United States has seen rapid evolution in attitudes and practices about
death and dying over the last several decades, beginning with the early
legal recognition in the *California Natural Death Act* (1976) of a patient's
right to refuse life-prolonging treatment in the face of terminal illness,
expanding in increased public awareness of issues of personal autonomy
in dying, raised by Derek Humphrey's how-to book of lethal drug
dosages, *Final Exit,* and blossoming in new sensitivity to physician roles
in aiding dying, both in the maverick social activism of Dr. Jack
Kevorkian and a New York grand jury's refusal to indict the respected
physician Timothy Quill. This process of cultural evolution has reached
legal recognition: in 1997, the U.S. Supreme Court jointly decided the
cases *Washington v. Glucksberg* and *Vacco v. Quill,* and while it held that
physician-assisted suicide is not a constitutional right, it also left states
free to make their own laws in this matter. Indeed, Oregon has made it
legal for a physician to provide a terminally ill patient who requests it
with a prescription for a lethal drug, thus bringing above ground the
practical manifestation of a long process of cultural change.

Cultural change like this draws on many factors, including changes in
medical technology, the epidemology of death, and the social and
legislative recognition of civil and personal rights in many other areas. Of
course, cultural change is not unidirectional. Although Oregon legalized
physician-assisted suicide, Maryland, among others, made it a felony.[2]
But it is possible to discern a pattern of increasing attention to end-of-life
issues and, I believe, to the issue of individual self-determination in the
matter of dying.

Loretta M. Kopelman and Kenneth A. De Ville (eds.), Physician-Assisted Suicide, 187–201.
© 2001 *Kluwer Academic Publishers. Printed in Great Britain.*

The story will not end here. This is the most important fact about cultural change – the fact that it is an ongoing process, one which we view only from some intermediate point. What I want to explore in this paper is the prospect of cultural change in the future, and the possibility that physician-assisted suicide may come to look very, very different from the desperation move that it is taken to be now.

1. THE WAY IT LOOKS NOW

Observe the current debate over physician-assisted suicide: on the one side, supporters of legalization appeal to the principle of autonomy, or self-determination, to insist that terminally ill patients have the right to extricate themselves from pain and suffering and to control as much as possible the ends of their lives. On the other, opponents resolutely insist on various religious, principled, or slippery-slope grounds that physician-assisted suicide cannot be allowed, because it is sacreligious, immoral, or poses risks of abuse. As vociferous and politicized as these two sides of the debate have become, however, proponents and opponents (tacitly) agree on a core issue: that the patient may choose to avoid suffering and pain. They disagree, it seems, largely about the means the patient and his or her physician may use to do so.

They also disagree about the actualities of pain control. Proponents of legalization insist that currently available forms of pain and symptom control are grossly inadequate and unsatisfactory. Citing such data as the SUPPORT study (1995)[3] they point to high rates of reported pain among terminally ill patients, inadequately developed pain-control therapies, physicians' lack of training in pain-control techniques, and obstacles and limitations to delivery of pain-control treatment, including restrictions on narcotic and other drugs. Pain and the suffering associated with other symptoms just aren't adequately controlled, proponents of legalization insist, so the patient is surely entitled to avoid them – if he or she so chooses – by turning to humanely assisted dying.

Many opponents of legalization, in contrast, insist that these claims are uninformed. Effective methods of pain control include timely withholding and withdrawal of treatment, sufficient use of morphine or other drugs for pain (even at the risk of foreseen, through unintended, shortening of life), and the discontinuation of artificial nutrition and hydration. When all other measures to control pain and suffering fail, there is always the possibility of terminal sedation: the induction of coma with concomitant withholding of nutrition and hydration, which, though it results in death, is not to be seen as killing.

Proponents of assisted suicide laugh at this claim. Terminal sedation, they retort, like the overuse of morphine, is functionally equivalent to causing death.

Despite these continuing disagreements about the effectiveness, availability, and significance of current pain control, both proponents and opponents in the debate appear to agree that *if* adequate pain control were available, there would be far less call for physician-assisted suicide. This claim is both predictive and normative. *If* adequate pain control were available, both sides argue, then physician-assisted suicide would be and should be quite infrequent – a "last resort," as Timothy Quill puts it, to be used only in exceptionally difficult cases when pain control really does fail. Borrowing an expression used by President Clinton to describe his view of abortion, most proponents insist that physician-assisted suicide should be "safe, legal, and rare." Likewise, opponents do not believe that it should be legal, but they also think that if it cannot be suppressed altogether or if a few very difficult cases remain, it should be very, very rare. The only real disagreement between opponents and proponents concerns those cases in which adequate pain control cannot be achieved.

What accounts for the opposing sides' underlying agreement that physician-assisted suicide should be rare is, I think, an unexamined assumption they share. This assumption is the view that the call for physician-assisted suicide is what might be called a *phenomenon of discrepant development:* a symptom of the disparity in development between two distinct capacities of modern medicine, the capacity to extend or prolong life and the capacity to control pain. Research, development, and delivery of technologies for the prolongation of life have raced far ahead; those for control of pain lag far behind. It is this situation of discrepant development that has triggered the current concern with physician-assisted suicide and the volatile public debate over whether to legalize it or not.

These opposing sides also recommend two simultaneous strategies: first, cutting back on overzealous prolongation of life (as Dan Callahan, for example, has long recommended (1987, 1993)), and second (as the hospice movement and others have been insisting (Foley, 1995))[4], accelerating the development of technologies for more effective methods of pain control, modes of delivery, and physician training. As life prolongation is held back a bit, pain control developments can "catch up," and the current situation of discrepant development between the two can be alleviated. Thus, calls for physician-assisted suicide can be expected to become rarer and rarer, and as medicine's capacities for pain control are finally equalized with its capacities for life prolongation, finally to virtually disappear. Almost no one imagines that there will not still be a few difficult situations in which life is prolonged beyond the point at which pain can be effectively controlled, but these will be increasingly infrequent, it is assumed, and in general, as the disparity between our capacities for life prolongation and for pain control shrinks, interest in and need for physician-assisted suicide will decrease and all but disappear.

Fortunately, this view continues, the public debate over physician-assisted suicide now so intense will not have been a waste, since it has both warned against the potential cruelty of overzealous prolongation of life and at the same time stimulated greater attention to imperatives of pain control. The current debate serves as social pressure for bringing equalization of the disparity about. Yet as useful as this debate is, this view holds, it will soon subside and disappear; we're just currently caught in a turbulent – but fleeting – maelstrom.

2. THE LONGER VIEW

That's how things look now. But I think we can also see our current concern with physician-assisted suicide in a longer-term, historically informed view. Consider just three of the many profound changes that affect matters of how we die. First, there has been a shift, beginning in the middle of the last century, in the ways in which human beings characteristically die. Termed the "epidemiological transition,"[5] this change involves a shift away from death due to parasitic and infectious disease (ubiquitous among humans in all parts of the globe prior to about 1850) to death in later life of degenerative disease – especially cancer and heart disease, which together account for almost two-thirds of deaths in the developed countries. This means dramatically extended lifespans and also deaths from diseases with characteristically extended downhill terminal courses. Second, there have been changes in religious attitudes about death: people are less likely to see death as divine punishment for sin, or to see suffering as a prerequisite for the afterlife, or to see suicide as a highly stigmatized and serious sin rather than the product of mental illness or depression. Third among the major shifts in cultural attitudes that affect the way we die is the increasing emphasis on the notion of individual rights of self-determination, reinforced in the latter part of this century by the civil rights movement's attention to individuals in vulnerable groups: this shift has affected self-perceptions and attitudes towards the terminally ill, and patients, including dying patients, are now recognized to have a wide array of rights previously eclipsed by the paternalistic practices of medicine.

These three transitions, along with many other concomitant cultural changes, invite us to see our current concern with physician-assisted suicide in a quite different light – not just as a phenomenon resulting from the currently disparate development of life-prolonging and pain-controlling technologies, a temporary anomaly, but as a precursor, an early symptom of a much more substantial sea-change in attitudes about death. We might call this shift in attitudes a shift towards "directed dying," or "self-directed dying," in which the individual who is dying plays a far more prominent, directive role than in earlier eras in determining how and when his or her death shall occur. In this changed view, dying is no longer *something that happens to you* but *something you do.*

To be sure, this shift – if it is one – can be seen as already well under way. Taking its legally visible start with the California Natural Death Act, terminally ill patients have already gained dramatically enlarged rights of self-determination in matters of guiding and controlling their own deaths, including rights to refuse treatment, discontinue treatment, stipulate treatment to be withheld at a later date, designate decision-makers, and to negotiate with their physicians, or have their surrogates do so, regarding such matters as DNR orders, withholding and withdrawal of ventilators, surgical procedures, nutrition and hydration, the use of opioids, and even terminal sedation. Some patients also negotiate, or attempt to negotiate, physician-assisted suicide or physician-performed euthanasia with their physicians. In all of these developments, we already see the patient playing a far more prominent role than in the past in determining the course of his or her dying process and its character and timing, and far more willingness on the part of physicians, family members, the law, and other parties to respect the patient's preferences and choices in these matters.

But this may be just the tip of a looming iceberg. For we may ask whether, much as we human beings have very recently made dramatic gains in control over our own reproduction (the birth control pill was introduced just thirty years ago), we are likewise beginning to make dramatic gains in control over our own dying, particularly in the last several decades. We cannot keep from dying altogether, of course. But by using directly caused death, as in physician-assisted suicide, it is possible to control many of dying's features: its timing in the downhill course of a terminal disease, its place, the exact agents which cause it, its observers, and so on. Indeed, as Robert Kastenbaum has argued, because it makes it possible to control the time, place, manner and people present at one's death, assisted suicide may very well become the *preferred* manner of dying (Kastenbaum, 1976).

But this conjecture does not yet show what could actually motivate such substantial social change, away from a culture which sees dying primarily as *something that happens to you*, to a culture which sees it as *something you do* – a deliberate, planned activity, one's final and culminative activity. What might do this, I think, is a conceptual change, or, more exactly, a shift in decisional perspective in choice-making about pain, suffering, and other elements of dying. It is the kind of shift in decisional perspective that evolves on a society-wide scale as a populace gains understanding of and control over a matter, a shift in choice-making perspective from a stance we might describe as immediately involved or "enmeshed," to one that is distanced and reflective. (I will use two Latin names for these stances later.) This shift can occur for many features of human experience – it has already largely occurred in the developed world with respect to reproduction – but it has not yet occurred with respect to dying. Rather, perhaps it has only just begun.

Take a patient, an average man. This particular man is so average that he just happens to have contracted that disease which is the usual diagnosis (as we know from the Netherlands)[6] in cases of physician-assisted suicide – cancer. He is also so average that this disease will kill him at just the average life-expectancy for males in the U.S., 72.8 years. Furthermore, he is so average that if he does turn to physician-assisted suicide, he will choose to forgo just about the same amount of life that, on average, Dutch patients receiving euthanasia or physician-assisted suicide do, less than 3.3 weeks (Emanuel and Battin, 1998). He has been considering physician-assisted suicide since his illness was first diagnosed (since he is an average man, this was about 29.6 months ago), but now, as his condition deteriorates, he thinks more seriously about it. His motivation includes both preemptive elements, the desire to avoid some of the very worst things that terminal cancer might bring him, and reactive elements, the desire to relieve some of the symptoms and other suffering that he is already experiencing. "It's bad enough now," he tells his doctor, "and it will probably get worse." He asks his doctor for the pills. He is perfectly aware of what he may miss – a number of weeks of continued life, the possibility of an unexpected cure, the chance, even if it is a longshot, of spontaneous regression or remission, and – not to be overlooked – the possibility that the worst is over, so to speak, and that the remainder of his downhill course in terminal cancer will not be so bad. He is also well aware that even a bad agonal phase may nevertheless include moments of great intimacy and importance with his family or friends. But he makes what he sees as a rational choice, seeking to balance the risks and possible benefits of easy death now, versus a little more continued life with a greater possibility of a hard death. He is making his choice *in medias res*, in the middle of things, as the physical, social, and emotional realities of terminal illness engulf him. He is enmeshed in his situation, caught in it, trapped between what seem like two bad alternatives – suffering, or suicide.

But, of course, he might have done his deciding about how his life shall end and whether to elect physician-assisted suicide in preference to the final stages of terminal illness from a quite different, more distanced perspective, a secular version of the view *sub specie aeternitatis*. This is not just an objective, depersonalized view – anybody's view – but his own, distinctively personal view not confined to a specific timepoint.[7] Rather than assessing his prospects from the point of view he has at the time at which he would continue or discontinue his life – that point late in the course of his illness when things have already become "bad enough" and are likely to get worse – he might have done his deciding, albeit rather more hypothetically, from the perspective of a more generalized view of his life. From this alternative perspective, what he would have seen is the overall shape of his life, and it is with respect to this that he would have made his choices about how it shall end. Of course, he could not know in advance whether he will contract cancer, or succumb to heart disease, or be hit by a bus – though he does know that he will die sometime or other. Consequently, his choices are necessarily conditional in form, "*if* I get cancer, I'll refuse aggressive treatment and use hospice care," "*if* I get AIDS, I'll ask for physician-assisted suicide," "*if* I get

Alzheimer's, I'll commit suicide on my own, since no physician besides Jack Kevorkian would help me," and so on. Although conditional in form and predicated on circumstances that may not occur, these may be real choices nonetheless, and, particularly because they are reiterated and repeated over the course of a lifetime, have real motive force.

The difference, then, between these two views is substantial. In the first, our average man with an average terminal cancer, deciding *in medias res*, is deciding whether or not to take the pills his physician has given him now. It is his last possible couple of weeks or a month (on average, 3.3 weeks) that he is deciding about. Even if continuing life threatens pain and other suffering, it is still all he has left, and while it may be difficult to live this life – all he has left – it may also be very difficult to relinquish it.

In contrast, if our average man were doing his deciding *sub specie aeternitatis*, from a distanced though still personal viewpoint not tied to a specific moment in his life, he would have been deciding all along between two different conceptions of his own demise, between two possible lives for himself. One of his possible lives would, on average, be 72.8 years long, the average lifespan for a male in the U.S., with the possibility of substantial suffering at the end – on average, as the SUPPORT study finds, a 50% chance, if conscious, of moderate to severe pain at least 50% of the time during the last three days before his death. The other of his possible lives would be about 72.7 years long, foreshortened on average 3.3 weeks by physician-assisted suicide, but with a markedly reduced possibility of substantial suffering at the end. (This shortening of the lifespan is not age-based but time-to-death based, planned for, on average, 3.3 weeks before an unassisted death would have occurred; it occurs in this example at age 72.7 just because our man is so average.) This latter, shortened life also offers our average man the opportunity to control the timing, the place, the manner, and so on of his death in the way he likes. Viewed *sub specie aeternitatis*, at any or many earlier points in one's life or from a vantage point standing outside life, so to speak, the difference between 72.8 and 72.7 seems negligible: these are both lives of average length not interrupted by grossly premature death. Why not choose the one in which the risk of agonal pain – as high as 50/50, if he is conscious, according to the SUPPORT study – is far, far less great, and the possibility of conscious, culminative personal experience, surrounded by family members, trusted friends, and permitting final prayers and good-byes, is far, far greater?

It may seem difficult to distinguish these two choices in practice. This is because we typically make our decisions about death and dying *in medias res*, not *sub specie aeternitatis*, and our medical practices, our bioethics discussions, and our background culture strongly encourage this. The call for assisted dying, like other patient pleas, is seen as a reaction to the circumstances of dying, not a settled, longer term, preemptive preference (Prado, 1990). True, some independently-minded individuals consider these issues in a kind of background, hypothetical way throughout their lives, but this is certainly not the practical norm. It would necessitate a substantial cultural shift from our current perspective.

But if this shift occurs, a slightly abbreviated lifespan in which there is dramatically reduced risk of pain and suffering will not only seem to be preferable to one which is negligibly longer but carries substantial risk of pain and suffering in its agonal phase, but it will also be seen as rational and normal to plan for this abbreviated lifespan and devise the means of bringing it about. A way to ensure such a demise, of course, is to plan for direct termination of life by assisted suicide. After all, one cannot count on being able to discontinue some life-prolonging treatment or other – refusing antibiotics, disconnecting a respirator – to hasten death and thus avoid what might be the worst weeks at the end. From this distanced perspective, a 72.7-year life with a virtually assured good end looks much, much better than a 72.8-year life that has an even chance of coming to a bad end. Arguably, it would be rational for any individual, except those for whom religious commitments or other scruples rule out suicide altogether, to plan to ensure this eventuality. But if it looks this way to one individual, it may also look this way to many others. It is thus plausible to imagine that physician-assisted suicide would not be rare, but rather a choice viewed as rational and preemptively prudent by many or even most members of the culture. Thus, it may come to be seen as a normal course of action, not a rarity or a "last resort." To be sure, there are other ways of abbreviating a lifespan to avoid terminal suffering – withdrawing or withholding treatment, overusing of morphine or other pain-relieving drugs, discontinuing artificial nutrition and hydration, and terminal sedation – but these cannot be used unless the patient's condition has already worsened and thus likely to involve that pain or suffering the person might choose to avoid. Thus these other modalities function primarily reactively; it is assisted suicide that can function preemptively.

But, as soon as planning for a normal, slight abbreviation in the lifespan by means of assisted suicide becomes conceptually possible not just for our hypothetical average man but for actual persons in general, it also becomes possible to imagine a wide range of context-specific cultural practices which might emerge surrounding physician-assisted suicide. After all, such a person understands and expects his lifespan to be one which will end in an assisted death a few weeks before he might otherwise have died; he can decide while he is still conscious, alert, and capable of deciding what location he wants it to take place in, what family members, caregivers, clergy, or others he wants to have present, what ceremonies, religious or symbolic, he wants conducted, etc. This suggests that more general social practices might grow up around these possibilities. After all, our average man sees his life this way; but it is possible for him to do this partly because the others in his society see their lives this way as well. Attitudes about death are heavily socially conditioned, and so are the perspectives from which choice-making about death is seen.

This is the precondition for the development of a whole range of social practices supporting such choices. These might include various kinds of practical supports, such as legal, insurance, and other policies which treat assisted dying as acceptable and normal; various sorts of cultural and religious practices which similarly treat assisted dying as acceptable and normal (for instance by developing rituals and rites concerning the forthcoming death); familial supports within the family, including family gatherings, preparing for the death, and sharing reminiscences and good-byes; pre-death dispositions of wills and life insurance (we already recognize viaticums, pre-death payoffs of life insurance for terminally ill patients); and even such now-inconceivable practices as pre-death funerals, understood as ceremonies of leave-taking and farewell, expressions of both celebration of a life complete and grief at its loss. In turn, such social practices may come to function as positive reasons for choosing a somewhat earlier, elective death – formerly and rudely called "physician-assisted suicide," even when pain control is no longer the issue at all. As a result, the new social pattern – so different from our current one – reinforces itself. This has nothing to do with a *Soylent Green* sort of view, in which people are forced into choices they do not genuinely make (this film can be understood only from our current, *in medias res* view); but a world in which their normal choices have genuinely changed, and changed for reasons which seem to them good.

Furthermore, if the culture-wide view of choice-making about death and dying were more fully held *sub specie aeternitatis* in this distanced, less enmeshed, and less reactive way, in which elective death becomes the norm, we could also expect the more frequent practice of "setting a date," as people who have contracted predictably terminal illnesses carry out the plans they had been developing all along for their own demises. Setting a date for one's own death – presumably, a couple of weeks or so before the date it might naturally have been, revisable of course in the light of any changes in the diagnosis or prognosis – would still be both preemptive and reactive in character, but far more preemptive than choices made *in medias res*, where choices will be highly reactive to the then-current circumstances the patient finds himself or herself in. The timing of such choices might always be revised in consultation with the physician; but what would be culturally reinforced would be the general commitment to advance planning for one's own death as well as a commitment to assuming a comparatively autonomist, directive role in it. Self-directed dying would be the norm, though of course different people would direct their deaths in quite different ways.

Profound changes affecting matters of how we die are already underway – the epidemiological transition, shifting from parasitic and infectious disease deaths to deaths of predictably degenerative disease; changes in religious conceptions of suicide so that it is not understood primarily as sin; and steadily increasing attention to patients' and terminally ill patients' rights of self-determination. It is an open conjecture whether this is where we may be going. Are we experiencing a mere temporary aberration in our basic cultural patterns of death and dying, an aberration which is a function of the discrepant development of technologies for life prolongation and for pain control? Or, are we seeing the first breaking waves of a sea-change from one perspective on death and dying to another, a far more autonomist and self-directive one?

Obviously, I can't say. But I can say that if this is what is happening, the assumption that physician-assisted suicide would or should be rare, an assumption still held by both sides in the current debate, will collapse. We would have no reason to assume that assisted dying should be rare, whatever the relationship between capacities for life prolongation and pain control. Of course, such a picture is very difficult to envision, since we do not think that way about death and dying now. But if we can at least see what is different about viewing personal choices about one's own death *sub specie aeternitatis* and in our current way, *in medias res,* enmeshed in particular circumstances, we can understand why cultural shift might occur.

Would it be a good thing, or a bad thing? I can hardly answer that question here, but let me close with a story I heard somewhere in the Netherlands several years ago. I do not remember the exact source of the story nor the specific dates or names, and it is certainly not representative of current practice in Holland. But it was told to me as a true story, and it went something like this.

Two friends, old sailing buddies, are planning a sailing trip in the North Sea in the summer. It is late February now, and they are discussing possible dates.

"How about July 21?" says Willem. "The North Sea will be calm, the moon bright, and there's a music festival on the southern coast of Denmark we could visit."

"Sounds great," answers Joost. "I'd love to get to the music festival. But I can't be gone then; the 21st is the date of my father's death."

"Oh, I'm so sorry, Joost," Willem replies. "I knew your father was ill. Very ill, with cancer. But I didn't realize he had died."

"He hasn't," Joost replies. "That's the day he will be dying. He's picked a date and made up his mind, and we all want to be there with him."

Such a story seems just that, a story, a fiction, somehow horrifying and also somehow liberating, but in any case virtually inconceivable to us. But it was not told to me as a fiction, but as a true story. In the foregoing discussion I've tried to explore the conceptual assumptions that might lie behind such a story, and consider whether in the future such stories might become more and more the norm. I have not tried to say whether this would be good or bad, but only that this might well be where we are going. In fact, I think it would be good – just as I think increasing personal control over reproduction is good – but I haven't argued for that view here.

Cultural change is an ongoing, long-term process of evolution, one which it is often hard to discern from a particular point in time. We see evolution in the past; but we have few tools to think about the future. I have tried to suggest that our current point of view about personal autonomy in death and dying is unduly limited. While we recognize that substantial change has already occurred, we fail to realize that change as great or greater may be coming in the future. Indeed, it could involve a full reversal of earlier cultural attitudes about one's own role in one's own death. Of course cultural change is not unidirectional, and there may be backward as well as forward motion. Nor do the attitudes of all members of a culture evolve at the same rate at the same time. Factors like wars, plagues, famines, scientific discoveries, and technological advances have reversed or hastened cultural change in the past, and could of course do so in the future. Just the same, I think it is possible to discern motion beyond the current view that physician-assisted suicide should and will be rare, a desperation move when nothing else works, toward the view that one's own death at the conclusion of terminal illness may be self-directed, that individuals can and should have the psychological and social freedom to reflect in a longer term way about their own future choices when they embark on the dying process, perhaps making physician-assisted suicide an eventual part of their plans, as well as the practical and legal freedom to plan whatever family gatherings, ceremonies, and religious observances they might wish – not as a desperate last resort or reactive escape from bad circumstances, but as a preemptively prudent, significant, culminative experience. How long this process of cultural change might take, and what might interrupt it or hasten it? Only time will tell.

University of Utah
Salt Lake City, Utah

NOTES

[1] This paper is a reframing of my "Physician-Assisted Suicide: Safe, Legal, Rare?", which appeared in Margaret P. Battin, Rosamond Rhodes, and Anita Silvers, eds., *Physician-Assisted Suicide: Expanding the Debate* (New York and London: Routledge, 1998).

[2] Editor's Note - In the 1990s over 20 bills were introduced in state legislatures to legalize PAS. All failed. In the same period, however, 16 states have passed laws explicitly prohibiting aid-in-dying bills.

[3] The SUPPORT Principal Investigators, in "A Controlled Trial to Improve Care for Seriously Ill Hospitalized Patients," (1995) show in a study of many hospitals that about 50% of dying hospitalized patients were reported to have experienced moderate to severe pain at least 50% of the time in their last three days of life.

[4] See especially the work of Kathleen Foley, in "Pain, physician-assisted suicide, and euthanasia," (1995) and other works.

⁵   The term originates with A.R. Omran, in "The Epidemiologic Transition: A Theory of the Epidemiology of Population Change," (1971), and the theory is augmented in A. Jay Olshansky and A. Brian Ault, "The Fourth Stage of the Epidemiologic Transition: The Age of Delayed Degenerative Disease," 1987.

[6]   Data on physician-assisted suicide and euthanasia in the Netherlands is provided by what is called the Remmelink Commission Report, found in an article by Paul J. van der Maas, Johannes J.M. van Delden, and Loes Pijnenborg, called "Euthanasia and other Medical Decisions Concerning the End of Life," (1992, and 1991); and the five-year update in Paul J. van der Maas, et al., in "Euthanasia, Physician-Assisted Suicide, and Other Medical Practices Involving the End of Life in the Netherlands, 1990–1995."

[7]   The distinction I am drawing here between personal views *in medias res* and *sub specie aeternitatis* is thus not quite the same as that drawn by Thomas Nagel between subjective and objective views, though it has much in common with Nagel's distinction in contexts concerning death. See Nagel's discussion in *The View from Nowhere* (1986), especially Chapter XI, section 3, on death.

REFERENCES

The SUPPORT Principal Investigators: 1995, 'A controlled trial to improve care for seriously ill hospitalized patients', *Journal of the American Medical Association* 274 (20) (1995): 1951–1998.

Callahan, D: 1987, *Setting Limits: Medical Goals in an Aging Society*, Simon and Schuster, New York, New York.

Callahan, D.: 1990, *What Kind of Life? The Limits of Medical Progress*, Simon and Schuster, New York, New York.

Callahan, D.: 1993, *The Troubled Dream of Life: Living with Mortality*, Simon and Schuster, New York, New York.

Emanuel, E.J. and Battin, M.P.: 1998, 'The economics of euthanasia: what are the potential cost savings from legalizing physician-assisted suicide?', *New England Journal of Medicine* 339(3), 167–172.

Foley, K.: 1995, 'Pain, physician-assisted suicide, and euthanasia', *Pain Forum* 4 (3) 128–131.

Kastenbaum, R.: 1976, 'Suicide as the preferred way of death', in E.S. Shneidman (ed.), *Suicidology: Contemporary Developments*, Grune & Stratton, New York, pp. 425–441.

Nagel, T.: 1986, *The View from Nowhere*, Oxford University Press, Oxford and New York, Chapter XI, section 3.

Omran, A.R.: 1971, 'The epidemiologic transition: a theory of the epidemiology of population change', *Milbank Memorial Fund Quarterly* 49 (4), 509–538.

Olshansky, A.J. and Ault, A.B.: 1987, 'The fourth stage of the epidemiologic transition: the age of delayed degenerative disease', in T.M. Smeeding et al., (eds.), *Should Medical Care Be Rationed By Age?* Rowman & Littlefield, Totowa, New Jersey, pp. 11–43.

Prado, C.G.: 1990, *The Last Choice: Preemptive Suicide in Advanced Age*, Greenwood Press, Westport, Connecticut.

Remmelink Commission Report, Paul J. van der Maas, Johannes J.M. van Delden, and Loes Pijnenborg: 1992, 'Euthanasia and other medical decisions concerning the end of life', published in full in English as a special issue of *Health Policy* 22, nos. 1 and 2 (1992), and, with Caspar W. N. Looman, in summary in *The Lancet* 338 (Sept. 14, 1991); 669–674; and the five-year update in Paul J. van der Maas, et al., 'Euthanasia, physician-assisted suicide, and other medical practices involving the end of life in the Netherlands', 1990–1995, *New England Journal of Medicine* 335(22):1699–1705 (1996).

WILLEM A. LANDMAN

A PROPOSAL FOR LEGALIZING ASSISTED SUICIDE AND EUTHANASIA IN SOUTH AFRICA

1. BACKGROUND

There is a serious initiative in South Africa (S.A.) to legalize physician-assisted suicide (PAS) and voluntary active euthanasia (VAE). In 1991, the S.A. Law Commission (the Commission) was requested to consider legislation regarding a "living will." This is a statutory[1] advisory body, appointed by the President, whose aim is the continuing renewal and improvement of South African law. It agreed to hear this request, but expanded its task to include the whole spectrum of end-of-life health-care decision-making issues, including physician-assisted suicide and voluntary active euthanasia.

Although I support this initiative on moral (Landman 1997; 1998) and constitutional grounds, there are controversial issues, some unique to S.A. and others of a more universal kind, which need to be addressed in the S.A. public debate and legislative process. The purpose of this paper is to suggest for discussion and critically comment on some of these issues. Before doing so, I first set out the essence of the Commission's arguments and proposals with respect to physician-assisted suicide and voluntary active euthanasia.

In 1997, the Commission published a "Discussion Paper" (SALC, 1997)[2] that sets out and comments on the legal position regarding end-of-life health-care decision-making in other countries. This Paper incorporates an omnibus end-of-life Draft Bill with clauses on refusal, withholding and withdrawal of life support, palliative care, advance directives, physician-assisted suicide and voluntary active euthanasia, and the powers of physicians and of the courts.

The Discussion Paper and its Draft Bill are likely to play an important role in framing the public debate. This Draft Bill suggested in the Discussion Paper would have to pass through several stages before it could become law. First, the Commission has already tested public opinion by requesting submissions that address explicitly posed questions regarding clauses in the Draft Bill. Next, the Commission would publish a Final Report and Draft Bill, which will then form the basis for likely public hearings by a Parliamentary Committee. Finally, this Committee may report to the S.A. Parliament, which would debate and approve or reject the bill. If it were approved, it would then pass to the President to reject it, or sign the bill making it law.

Whether the S.A. Parliament will, at the conclusion of this process, actually legalize physician-assisted suicide and voluntary active euthanasia is an open question. Given the growing sense that the 1996 Constitution's justiciable Bill of Rights,[3] rather than sectional moral or religious convictions, should inform public debate and legal reform, it will not be surprising if S.A. adopts the world's first comprehensive end-of-life health-care decision-making statute.[4]

Although the Commission's Draft Bill addresses all end-of-life medical decision-making, including involuntary and non-voluntary euthanasia,[5] I limit my brief summary of its arguments and proposals to the question of legalizing physician-assisted suicide and voluntary active euthanasia.

The Commission argues that it is necessary to investigate the moral case for legalizing physician-assisted suicide and voluntary active euthanasia since there is a "relatively small percentage of mentally competent patients who are terminally ill, for whom no effective medical treatment is available and for whom the palliative medical skills are not adequate. They may be subject to unbearable pain or discomfort despite all the known techniques and not prepared to continue living under such circumstances" (3.33).[2,6] The Draft Bill defines "terminal illness" as "all illness, injury or other physical or mental conditions which (a) will inevitably result in the death of the patient concerned within a relatively short time and which is causing the patient extreme suffering; or (b) is causing the patient to be in a persistent and irreversible vegetative condition [PVS] with the result that no meaningful existence is possible for the patient" (SALC, 1997).

The Commission's position argues that unless a genuine distinction, moral or legal, can be made between physician-assisted suicide and voluntary active euthanasia, they should be treated in the same way in the Draft Bill (3.78). They are both, legally speaking, versions of "active euthanasia" since in both cases the person to whom the request is directed performs the act, and the intention in both cases is to cause death (3.78). At issue is the *principle of assistance in the ending of life*, or voluntary euthanasia (3.78). The key question according to the Commission is "whether our community [SA] would consider a request for euthanasia as reasonable or unreasonable where the consent is given by a mentally competent person with full knowledge and understanding of the extent, nature and consequences of his or her consent" (3.79).

Should the public and parliament, after debate, support the enactment of physician-assisted suicide and voluntary active euthanasia legislation, the Commission proposes a clause be included in the enabling legislation (Draft Bill, Section 5). This clause should stipulate that it shall not be unlawful for a physician requested by a patient "to make an end to the patient's suffering, or to enable the patient to make an end to his or her suffering by way of *administering* [voluntary active euthanasia] or *providing* [physician-assisted suicide] some or other lethal agent" (3.91, my italics), provided all the following conditions are met: the patient (a) is terminally ill, (b) is subject to extreme suffering, (c) is over 18 and mentally competent, (d) is adequately informed, (e) makes a request based on an informed and well considered decision, (f) has had an opportunity to re-evaluate his or her request but persists, and (g) has no other way to be released from suffering. Other safeguards relate to conferring with an independent physician, the maintenance of a written record, prohibiting persons other than physicians from terminating a patient's life, immunizing physicians against civil, criminal and disciplinary liability, and an opt-out conscience clause for physicians.

2. CONTROVERSIAL ISSUES

A. Ad hominem Responses

Worldwide, voluntary active euthanasia is hardly on the public-policy agenda. In the Netherlands, physician-assisted suicide and voluntary active euthanasia are not prosecuted, provided certain conditions are satisfied. Whereas physician-assisted suicide has been legal in the state of Oregon in the United States (U.S.) since October 27, 1997, it is no longer legal in the Northern Territory of Australia. Should the controversial S.A. initiative be carried through, it is likely to meet with a skeptical, even hostile, reception internationally, judging by some of the responses to the Northern Territory's physician-assisted suicide initiative. For example, the well-known U.S. medical ethicist, Arthur Caplan (1998, p. 225), called it a "whimper" from an "obscure" part of the world. Caplan (1998, p. 225) obfuscates the debate with his characterization of the Northern Territory's initiative: "The Northern Territory is the first legislative body since Hitler's Germany and Stalin's Russia to allow doctors to engage in euthanasia." This comment mischievously equates incomparable actions, associated only because the word "euthanasia" has different meanings, thereby cheapening the mindless suffering inflicted on victims of totalitarianism. The Nazis were motivated by neither mercy nor respect for autonomy, but rather by the goal of achieving the racial purity of the *Volk* (Kuhse, 1991, pp. 301–302). Thus, the Nazi analogy is wholly inapt. Significantly, research indicates that many survivors of the holocaust see no similarity between physician-assisted suicide, as contemplated in a purely medical context (which some of them indeed oppose), and the Nazi policy of legalized murder, euphemistically called "euthanasia" (Leichtentritt *et al.*, 1999).

The S.A. initiative would do well not to engage such *ad hominem* responses which employ faulty assumptions and analogies.

B. Legal Definitions and Underlying Values

Several definitions in the Draft Bill are clearly in need of clarification. The term "terminal illness" extends to persons (a) whose death will occur within a relatively short time and who are subject to extreme suffering, or (b) in a PVS. "Within a relatively short time" may be too vague. To reduce uncertainty, it may be preferable to replace it by "*within six months*" which is a more common and specific meaning. This leaves open the question whether physicians are capable of predicting accurately the time of death. Still, the six-month limit is less nebulous than "death within a relatively short time" and is more likely to rule out extremes that are either too short (such as a week or month) or too long (such as a year).

The University of Cape Town (U.C.T.) Bioethics Centre, whose members include prominent academic physicians, proposes that this legal definition of "terminal illness" included in the Commission's report be expanded to include a third category: persons who are chronically dependent on life support, since persistent organ failure is fatal in the absence of advanced life-support systems (Benatar et al., 1997, p. 2). The Bioethics Centre recommendation points out that such a broadening of the definition would not permit voluntary active euthanasia of those with chronic renal failure because they can lead a life of good quality. Such patients would not satisfy the Draft Bill's additional condition that the patient is subject to extreme suffering. However, making such general quality-of-life judgments, and special reference to chronic renal failure, appear inconsistent with the Bioethics Centre's recommendation that physician-assisted suicide and voluntary active euthanasia should be made available to some individuals who are not terminally ill. I now turn to that proposal.

The Bioethics Centre proposes that the term "terminal illness" be used disjunctively with the term "intractable and unbearable illness." If patients' end-of-life options, as envisaged by the Draft Bill, are grounded in respect for autonomy, then, according to the Bioethics Centre recommendations, "it would be arbitrary to permit these options only to those whose death was relatively close and deny it to those suffering chronic and degenerative conditions including multiple sclerosis, amyotrophic lateral sclerosis, motor-neurone disease and quadriplegia" (Benatar et al., 1997, p. 2). The Bioethics Centre report then proposes the following alternative definition: *"Intractable and unbearable illness" means a bodily disorder that (1) cannot be cured or successfully palliated, and (2) that causes such severe suffering that death is preferable to continued life* (Benatar et al., 1997, p. 2).

The inclusion of some non-terminal illnesses as a category for which patients might receive physician-assisted suicide or voluntary active euthanasia speaks to the fact that there are a number of medical conditions that cause extreme suffering, but are not terminal. Still, the Bioethics Centre definition raises an important question of interpretation. If a patient suffers from a *mental* or *dementing* disorder that does not render her mentally incompetent, is she capable, in theory, of suffering from an "intractable or unbearable disease" that grounds a legitimate request for assistance with dying? If so, does referring to an "intractable and unbearable illness" as a "bodily disorder" permit such an interpretation? Although all disorders have some bodily or physiological foundation, we tend to think of them as either physiological or psychological, so some may interpret the qualifier "bodily" as excluding mental or demanding disorders. Consequently, for the legal definition of "intractable and unbearable illness" to cover those sorts of cases, the term "bodily" should be removed, and the term "disorder" may have to be given a more precise, yet more comprehensive, definition. If suffering is understood as an emotional response to more than minimal pain *or distress*, then it can be either physical *or mental* (or both). But would the definition of "intractable or unbearable illness" include such a wide interpretation, namely, a disorder that may cause *mental suffering alone*? For the sake of clarity, either the term "physical or mental suffering" should be used, or the term "suffering" should be defined in the Draft Bill.

Extending the meaning of "illness" to encompass patients who may be neither terminal nor in (physical) pain is of course controversial and raises questions about the moral commitments underlying the debate about legalizing physician-assisted suicide and voluntary active euthanasia. Supporters of broader availability of physician-assisted suicide and voluntary active euthanasia can appeal to the values of autonomy and well being (Brock, 1992), which are recognized by being respectful of autonomous decisions and showing mercy (refraining from doing harm, or doing good). Some people die in circumstances where they autonomously request assistance with dying that will hasten death in ways other than terminal sedation,[6] namely, physician-assisted suicide or voluntary active euthanasia. For them the conceptual connection between life and good is broken if life irreversibly fails to come up to a minimum standard of basic human goods (Foot, 1977). Dying is a natural part of life, and mercy should therefore not be confined to restitution (curing, healing, or extending life) and palliative care, but should embrace the notion of life-shortening assistance with dying. Recognizing autonomy and well being in this ultimate context challenges what has become the traditional combative attitude to death in contemporary Western culture, that is, death as a failure, or something to be conquered, regardless of the quality of life and the impossibility of restitution. Taking autonomy and well being seriously entails reassessing and contextualizing the goals of medicine, given our inevitable destiny.

In addition to principled objections directed at this broad definition of "illness" and its implications for physician-assisted suicide and voluntary active euthanasia, others may arise from undercutting the belief that human life *as such* is intrinsically valuable. According to this view, anything that hastens death, including withholding or withdrawal of life support, may be regarded as intrinsically wrong, regardless of quality-of-life considerations or the subjective value assigned to life by the person whose life it is. As a result, the goals of medicine do not extend beyond restitution and palliative care. Yet another objection appeals not to principles, but to possible bad consequences, or slippery-slope abuses, that may follow from legalizing physician-assisted suicide and voluntary active euthanasia. (I address these in some detail below.)

In addition, the Bioethics Centre commentary contends that the term "euthanasia" should be defined since it is used in the Draft Bill, and proposes the following legal definition that would cover voluntary and non-voluntary euthanasia: *"The intentional bringing about of a being's death for that being's own sake"* (Benatar et al., 1997, p. 1). This definition is, however, too broad since it would also include withholding and withdrawal of life support, sometimes (unfortunately) called "passive euthanasia," which is clearly not the intention of the Draft Bill (compare Sections 3 and 5). In addition, since the Draft Bill proposes legalizing both physician-assisted suicide and voluntary active euthanasia, both being regarded as closely related instances of assistance with dying, while using only the term "euthanasia," the legal definition of "euthanasia" should cover both practices.

To avoid these lapses, I therefore propose the following definition: *"The intentional bringing about of an individual's death for that individual's own sake, where a positive act of a person other than that individual, and not merely withholding or withdrawal of life-sustaining treatment, is either a contributory cause or a proximate cause of death."* Alternatively, both the terms "physician-assisted suicide" and "voluntary active euthanasia" should be used and legally defined in the Draft Bill, respectively in terms of a contributory cause and a proximate cause. This definitional proposal is premised on a counterfactual analysis according to which an act or omission can be a (contributory) cause of death, or necessary in the circumstances (as with physician-assisted suicide), without being a proximate, direct, or last cause (as with voluntary active euthanasia) (Mackie, 1974). And a contributory cause figures in an analysis of intending death and responsibility for death.

Since there is a controversy as to whether administering artificial nutrition and hydration is a form of medical treatment, the formulation "medical treatment *or artificial nutrition and hydration*" should be used in the relevant clauses of the Draft Bill.

C. The Physician-Assisted Suicide/Voluntary Active Euthanasia Distinction

The Draft Bill deals with physician-assisted suicide and voluntary active euthanasia as one entity because the Commission believes that the central relevant issue is the principle of assistance with dying. The Commission's approach makes no distinction legally between ending a patient's suffering, and enabling a patient to make an end to her suffering.

This is a crucial aspect of the proposed legislation. Equating physician-assisted suicide and voluntary active euthanasia would probably find little intellectual support in countries like the U.S. where opponents as well as proponents of physician-assisted suicide believe that there is a moral barrier between physician-assisted suicide and voluntary active euthanasia, with the latter being less justifiable (Battin, 1991; Quill et al., 1992). Although the supporters of the S.A. Draft Bill should expect strong criticism in this regard, the claim that there is a general moral difference between the two is still weak (Dixon, 1998). There are three broad grounds on which one could attempt to drive a moral wedge between physician-assisted suicide and voluntary active euthanasia, namely, (a) causation, intention, and moral responsibility, (b) possible bad consequences or slippery-slope abuses, and (c) physicians' general (natural) duties and specific (professional) moral obligations, and the goals of medicine. None of these supports a *general* moral difference, such that any instance of physician-assisted suicide would be morally preferable to any instance of voluntary active euthanasia.

For two reasons it may be difficult to demonstrate general moral differences between physician-assisted suicide and voluntary active euthanasia on these grounds. First, a suggested distinction may fail to carry the *moral burden* placed on it. For example, the bare fact that a physician is not a proximate cause of death, as with physician-assisted suicide and unlike voluntary active euthanasia, does not rule out that her action causally contributed to the death, nor that she did not intend it, nor that she is absolved from moral responsibility. Second, morally relevant differences may be determined in the "thickness" of a *particular context*, while the mere fact that an action is an instance of physician-assisted suicide rather than voluntary active euthanasia is not as such a moral determinant. For example, both physician-assisted suicide and voluntary active euthanasia may or may not lead to bad consequences. Also, obligations to respect autonomy and be merciful may require that a physician performs either physician-assisted suicide or voluntary active euthanasia, depending on contingent circumstances, or how these obligations are conceived, or what the goals of medicine are believed to be. Positively, if physician-assisted suicide and voluntary active euthanasia are regarded as morally equivalent, other things being equal, physicians will not have to abandon those patients for whom voluntary active euthanasia is the best option, or be instruments in their ongoing suffering, but will be able to facilitate a good death when continued life is worse than death.

Even if one denies a general *intrinsic* moral difference between voluntary active euthanasia and physician-assisted suicide, one could still argue that there is an important *evidentiary* difference between the two, and, consequently, that the distinction could have some value in practice. Thus, the Bioethics Centre has argued that physician-assisted suicide is a better test of the voluntariness of the choice to die, or of the patient's resolve to end his or her life (Benatar et al., 1997, pp. 3–4). The Bioethics Centre recommends that voluntary active euthanasia not be permitted where physician-assisted suicide is an option. This restriction, however, may ask too much of suffering patients. Instead of stipulating such an absolute condition, it would be preferable to acknowledge a strong, but rebuttable, presumption that physician-assisted suicide is preferable to voluntary active euthanasia. This respects autonomy and constitutes appropriate assistance with dying for patients who fear abandonment, or who simply prefer not to commit suicide. Moreover, given certain physical incapacities, such as quadriplegia or the inability to swallow, fairness requires the availability of voluntary active euthanasia as an option.

In fact, since the right to equality in the S.A. Constitution's Bill of Rights prohibits unfair discrimination by the state against anyone on the grounds of disability, it seems likely that the exclusion of voluntary active euthanasia as an option would constitute *unfair discrimination* against the physically disabled.[7] Limiting suffering patients' options to physician-assisted suicide would unfairly favor persons who are physically able to take their own lives, in effect allowing those who suffer grievously to kill themselves, but barring those who are so debilitated that they cannot do it themselves. Hence, physician-assisted suicide and voluntary active euthanasia are complementary and seem inextricably bound together by the S.A. Constitution.

D. Assisters of Suicide and Performers of Voluntary Active Euthanasia

The Draft Bill states that only physicians ("medical practitioners") should be legally empowered to assist with suicide and perform voluntary active euthanasia. The Bioethics Centre, however, recommends that physicians should not be the only persons empowered to assist with dying, but that close family (such as spouses, adult children, or parents) or friends should also be permitted to do so (Benatar et al., 1997, pp. 4–5). The Draft Bill's limitation in this regard, in Section 5(4), is seen as an unnecessary interference with liberty, redundant in view of other procedural safeguards, and problematic because dying is a lonely event which should be mitigated by the comfort drawn from close personal relationships. The Bioethics Centre believes that locating assistance with dying in such a wider context of caring may counter the perception of a close connection between death and physicians, and erosion of trust in the medical profession.

There are two main approaches. Either physicians, who make factual determinations as required by procedural safeguards, remain in full control of all aspects of assistance with dying, or persons other than physicians may also be legally empowered to assist with dying in limited ways. Whichever approach is adopted, physicians, since they are the only persons in S.A. suitably qualified and licensed to prescribe drugs necessary for terminating life, should be the only persons allowed to make *essential clinical determinations* (diagnoses, prognoses, outlining clinical options) and *prescribe drugs*.

Patients, however, increasingly choose to die at home where they are cared for by loved ones. Should they choose assisted suicide or voluntary active euthanasia, they may wish to be assisted by those who are closest to them. Although evidence is sketchy and incomplete, it is an open secret such assistance is rendered, in S.A. and around the world. Should assisted suicide by laypersons become law in S.A., additional procedural safeguards need to ensure that assisters of suicide and performers of voluntary active euthanasia are knowledgeable about *methods* of assistance with dying. Of course, physicians will have to be vigilant about possible conflicts of interest between family members and the patient, as well as disagreements among family members, but these same cautions apply currently to withholding or withdrawal of life support.

If persons other than physicians are legally empowered to assist with dying, other caregivers, such as nurses or aides, should also be permitted to assist with suicide or perform voluntary active euthanasia. Moreover, with the inclusion of traditional healers in health-care delivery, it is conceivable that they, too, may feel entitled to assist with dying. However, if any layperson were to be legally empowered to assist, it is essential that their participation be linked to *actual administration* (such as handing over pills or giving a lethal injection), and not making clinical determinations or prescribing drugs.

E. Competent Minors' Requests for Physician-Assisted Suicide and Voluntary Active Euthanasia

The Draft Bill also raises the controversial but neglected issue whether legislation should recognize a right of competent minors (persons under 18) to choose physician-assisted suicide or voluntary active euthanasia (or to issue advance directives in this regard). Should we presume that minors cannot be the best judges of whether physician-assisted suicide or voluntary active euthanasia is in their own best interest, and that parents or guardians should have complete decision-making authority?

With older children and adolescents chronological age becomes a less accurate indicator of mental competence. Mental competence means having the required decision-making ability, that is, abilities of communication, understanding, reflective deliberation, and judgment, to make a particular kind of decision (Brock, 1987). Minors are no doubt competent to make all sorts of medical decisions, and this is acknowledged by the law. S.A. abortion law, for example, recognizes the mental competence of minors to make serious medical decisions by requiring consent for abortion only from the pregnant woman, who is defined as "any female person of any age."[8] Moreover, the issue of children's legal competence is currently under review in S.A. The S.A. Law Commission (SALC, 1998), in its review of the *Child Care Act*,[9] and addressing the issue of children's informed consent for medical treatment or surgical intervention, asks whether the arbitrary (legal) age limits set in this regard are (morally) appropriate.

Are minors competent to make their own health-care decisions even if these may hasten death? There is no general answer to this question, because it involves borderline issues about a particular individual's level of mental development or maturity, and this may be greatly influenced by prolonged experience of repeated hospitalization, treatment for terminal illness, and suffering. Some commentators argue persuasively that minors suffering from, for example, end-stage renal disease (Doyal et al., 1994) or terminal cancer (Freyer, 1992), and who possess the required cognitive and emotional wherewithal, should have the right to refuse life-sustaining treatment. It follows that if physician-assisted suicide and voluntary active euthanasia are legalized some mature older minors should also have the right to choose these life-shortening options for themselves.

Minors are, however, under the legal decision-making authority of their parents, and parents are presumed to do what is in the best interest of their children. Clearly, parents are best suited to make decisions for incompetent minors, but mentally competent minors are a special case and parents should respect their capacity for self-determination and their considered choices in pursuit of their well-being or best interest, even if it means that their lives are shortened.

Thus, a convincing case might be made for competent minors' legal entitlement to physician-assisted suicide and voluntary active euthanasia (or refusal of life-sustaining treatment), on the grounds of respect for personal autonomy, mercy, and justice. Legislation may require additional procedural safeguards, addressing such issues as mentally competent minors' decision-making capacity, respecting parents' or guardians' authority by involving them intimately in all deliberation throughout the decision-making process (Wharton et al., 1996) and requiring their consent, written certification by a psychiatrist, registered clinical psychologist, or social worker, personally familiar with the circumstances of the particular patient, and the power of the courts to grant minors' wishes against those of their parents in highly exceptional and compelling circumstances.

F. Constitutional Justifications for Legalization

The question whether physician-assisted suicide and voluntary active euthanasia are morally justifiable practices is, of course, separate from the question whether they should be legalized. Significantly, there are two constitutional reasons, peculiar to S.A., why the question of legalizing physician-assisted suicide and voluntary active euthanasia will need to be addressed sooner or later.

First, the S.A. Constitution's Bill of Rights includes potentially conflicting rights. Whereas it could be argued that physician-assisted suicide and voluntary active euthanasia may violate the constitutional right to life, this right is not absolute and has to be weighed against other constitutional rights,[3] such as the right to "freedom and security of the person," and specifically the right "not to be deprived of freedom arbitrarily or without just cause," and the right of "control over [one's] body." Moreover, "the [S.A.] Constitution speaks of a right to life, but not of a duty to live. Given their conceptual logic, rights may be waived. If continued life is no longer in somebody's interest that person should be free to waive the right to life" (Benatar et al., 1997, p. 3).

Second, a recent ruling by S.A.'s Constitutional Court in the *Soobramoney*[10] case has the effect that the state, in certain circumstances, may be inconsistent if it denies a request for physician-assisted suicide or voluntary active euthanasia.[11] The appellant, in the final stages of chronic renal failure, claimed that he was entitled to emergency dialysis, given the constitutional right to life and provision that no-one may be refused emergency medical treatment. The court rejected his application on the grounds that withholding life-prolonging treatment, or rationing care, is compatible with a constitutional human-rights approach, given scarce resources. Withholding dialysis, a scarce resource, led directly to the appellant's death. But given that the state can legitimately withhold resources necessary for life, it would be inconsistent, as well as cruel, if the state were also to deny the "condemned" man's request for physician-assisted suicide or voluntary active euthanasia so that he could die sooner and, perhaps, with less suffering. On what grounds can the state sanction death when it is a bad for the applicant, but deny it when it is a good, especially if the state has made death the only option?

G. Universal Slippery-Slope Considerations

The slippery-slope argument that legalized physician-assisted suicide and voluntary active euthanasia will lead to abuse or exploitation of the poor and vulnerable presents a case against legalizing these practices in any community. Considering the extensive international concern regarding slippery slope fears, the Commission should have devoted more consideration to this serious objection, and determined what it implies for procedural safeguards. Still, the slippery-slope argument, which has logical and empirical versions, is frequently overstated and speculative.

According to the *logical* version, the justification used for physician-assisted suicide and voluntary active euthanasia would also justify other forms of killing. Helga Kuhse (1991, p. 301) points out that it does not follow, on logical grounds, that the reasons justifying physician-assisted suicide and voluntary active euthanasia, namely, respect for autonomy and mercy, would also justify killings that are neither merciful nor respectful of autonomy. People routinely make a clear distinction between moral and immoral practices, even if they are closely related in other respects, including justified and unjustified forms of killing, for example, in self-defense or war. Moreover, there is no logical reason why physicians, even assuming they might sometimes wish their patients dead, will slide down a slippery slope only in respect of one subset of end-of-life decisions, namely, physician-assisted suicide and voluntary active euthanasia. It seems reasonable to assume that what is true of withholding or withdrawal of treatment, or terminal sedation, is *prima facie* also true of physician-assisted suicide and voluntary active euthanasia, that is, the slippery slope dangers would be equally existent or non-existent in either case.

Second, available *empirical* evidence does not show that ethically or legally justified assistance with dying leads, as a matter of fact, to unjustified killings (Kuhse, 1991, p. 301). I am unaware of evidence of abuse in respect of existing practices which hasten death, such as withholding or withdrawal of life support when a competent patient requests it, or terminating the life support of an incompetent terminally ill person without an advance directive, and available studies seem to imply that it does not (e.g., Turner et al., 1996).

The main source of evidence about a possible slippery slope in respect of both physician-assisted suicide and voluntary active euthanasia is the Netherlands, where these practices had not been criminally prosecuted, provided certain criteria were met, and were legalized early in 2001. In addition, physician-assisted suicide data from Oregon have recently become available (Chin et al., 1999). This Oregon study of the first full calendar year of legalized physician-assisted suicide (1998) shows no evidence of abuse, indicating that procedural safeguards are probably achieving their goal. However, others caution that these data may not tell the full truth (Foley and Hendin, 1999). Some critics argue that people in the Netherlands are sometimes "seduced" into death. Other commentators note that opponents of the Dutch practices misuse data and stretch arguments to make their cases (Dworkin, 1997; van der Maas et al., 1996; van der Wal et al., 1996). Defenders of the Dutch practice have provided data to support the degree to which safeguards have been implemented and contend that the Dutch experience should calm the anxieties of those who fear legalized euthanasia. Thus, it is not at all clear what Dutch data may mean for legalizing physician-assisted suicide and voluntary active euthanasia in S.A. Certainly, long-standing universal health care and well-developed social support programs in the Netherlands (Battin, 1990; 1993) make valid comparisons with S.A. (and the U.S.) difficult.

Moreover, the physician–patient relationship is more personal and stable in the Netherlands than in most countries, and money and medicine do not form the same problematic alliance that may exist in some other countries. Still, even if there were cases of abuse in the Netherlands, it does not follow that procedural safeguards in S.A. legislation will fail to provide adequate protection for poor and vulnerable patients (Dworkin, 1997, p. 43). It is the moral responsibility of proponents of legalization to see to it that they do provide essential safeguards. But it is equally the moral responsibility of opponents to show that having no legislation is the best way to prevent *status quo* abuse (Battin, 1992, p. 143).

More generally, if it is morally prohibited to legalize a practice unless absolute compliance is guaranteed, then we will have to ban practices like driving cars or the implementation of basic rights, like the right to free speech. Quite rightly, we do not curtail individuals' legitimate liberties because *others* may and do abuse them. All human endeavor, including the *status quo*, has the potential for abuse, and demanding (near) absolute guarantees diverts attention from substantive deliberation about what is the right thing to do.

Nevertheless, procedural safeguards in the Draft Bill may need to be tightened so that the aspects and time line of a request for assistance with dying are more explicit, without becoming overbearing. For example, an informed and well-considered decision, made known in the form of an oral request, should be followed by a waiting period of a stipulated number of days (seven, for example[12]). There should then be a written request followed by a second waiting period (48 hours, for example), and there should be repeated, formalized opportunities to rescind the decision.

H. Slippery-Slope Considerations in the South African Cultural Context

Legalizing physician-assisted suicide or voluntary active euthanasia may raise additional slippery-slope issues specific to the S.A. cultural context. Four kinds of considerations may call for more specific procedural safeguards, apart from ongoing transformation of the health-care system.

First, S.A. is a *multicultural society* with indigenous populations, traditional communities, and eleven official languages that make misunderstanding in personal communication a very real possibility. Patients should be able to discuss their options and considered choices without language being an impediment to their understanding. Where physicians are unable to communicate with patients in their first language, qualified interpreters should facilitate the process and certify that patients understand all aspects of their decision (MacFarlane, 1997). This, together with other procedural safeguards and professional oversight (SAHR, 1998: ch. 3), should address concerns about the potential for personal, professional and institutional abuse (Battin, 1992).

Second, many South Africans have *educational deficits* which will limit their ability to understand fully the meaning and implications of a legal right to physician-assisted suicide and voluntary active euthanasia. A general legal prohibition of physician-assisted suicide and voluntary active euthanasia, however, simply on the ground that "traditional" people may have peculiar difficulties of understanding, would be a paternalistic overreaction to the problem. Still, some may view legalizing physician-assisted suicide and voluntary active euthanasia as an imposition of Western values on people with different cultural belief systems (MacFarlane, 1997, p. 182). These options, however, are consistent with rights guaranteed by the S.A. Constitution, and they will not be imposed on anyone provided safeguards are respected. Nevertheless, the creation of a legal right to active assistance with dying, in the forms of physician-assisted suicide (or assisted suicide) and voluntary active euthanasia, will clearly impose new educational responsibilities on society.

Given fuller senses of community and family, different notions of respect and care for the elderly and sickly, as well as alternative values informing notions of health, disease and death in traditional communities, I suspect the demand for physician-assisted suicide and voluntary active euthanasia among traditional people will be extremely limited. With urbanization, however, comes increasing replacement of traditional communitarian values and practices with more individualistic ones, and, consequently, an increased need to expand end-of-life options.

Third, South Africans have hugely *differential access to scarce health-care resources*, and specific resources will be required to exercise a legal right to physician-assisted suicide and voluntary active euthanasia. The vast majority of patients in rural areas will not have routine access to a physician,[13] let alone two, as will be required by legalized physician-assisted suicide and voluntary active euthanasia, and will therefore be unable to choose these forms of assistance with dying. This is an issue of equity that has to be addressed in the transformation process to a national health service.

Although a study comparing treatment decisions in one Cape Town and one London ICU found little difference in the withholding and withdrawal of life-support technologies (Turner et al., 1996), some critics may argue that the risk of abuse in respect of legalized physician-assisted suicide and voluntary active euthanasia will be greater given the endemic scarcity of resources. This concern must be taken seriously, but given effective procedural safeguards, why should physician-assisted suicide and voluntary active euthanasia be singled out if withholding and withdrawal of life support likewise save scarce resources required to keep patients alive? Moreover, one could argue that it may be preferable for a patient, who meets all the criteria for physician-assisted suicide or voluntary active euthanasia, to know that there is an escape route when health-care insurance cover is exhausted, rather than having to suffer due to a combination of scarce resources and legal prohibition. Although this would appear to compromise the freedom of a physician-assisted suicide or voluntary active euthanasia request, is it fundamentally different (and morally more problematic) than other treatment or non-treatment decisions made in an environment of resource scarcity?

Fourth, some observers may believe that S.A., with its past of white-on-black *racial discrimination*, should be the last place in the world to legalize physician-assisted suicide or voluntary active euthanasia. These concerns, although understandable, need to take account of countervailing considerations. Procedural safeguards are directed at eliminating *all* forms of unjustified physician-assisted suicide and voluntary active euthanasia. Generally speaking, physicians are held in high esteem in S.A. and are ordinarily trusted to have the interests of their patients, black and white, at heart. The complicity of state-employed physicians in the state-sanctioned murder of black activist Steve Biko in 1977 is not the norm. New legislation allows for more effective control of the health professions through the exercise of expanded, including disciplinary, powers of the professional boards established for each of the health professions (SAHR, 1998: ch. 3). The overwhelming majority of the members of the S.A. Parliament are black. During the 1990s, admissions of black students to medical schools has increased significantly (SAHR, 1998: ch. 5), and the government is committed to addressing the remaining demographic imbalances. And, finally, there is little empirical evidence to suggest that end-of-life decisions are fundamentally different in S.A. Together, these considerations serve as counterweights to the argument that legalizing physician-assisted suicide and voluntary active euthanasia in S.A. will lead to abuse or a slide down a race-oriented slippery slope.

3. CONCLUSION

I hope there will be a serious debate in S.A. that avoids being held captive by alleged moral barriers – between withholding/withdrawal of treatment and physician-assisted suicide, or between physician-assisted suicide and voluntary active euthanasia – which are incapable of carrying the burden placed upon them. The S.A. initiative would do well to avoid the implicit assumption, often made in these debates, that physicians, but for the threat of criminal sanction, would eagerly dispose of the poor and the vulnerable. The challenge is to create the social and procedural conditions that will assist people to choose freely, autonomously, and in a caring environment the manner of their death, and to die with dignity, whether that means palliative care, terminal sedation, withholding or withdrawal of treatment, physician-assisted suicide, assisted suicide or voluntary active euthanasia.

4. POSTSCRIPT AND UPDATE

In August 1999, since the presentation of the foregoing discussion, the SALC published its final "Report" (SALC, 1999) containing a Draft Bill, modified in view of submissions from the public. It was submitted to the Minister of Justice, and will serve as the basis for further public discussion and Parliament's legislative process. The Draft Bill deals with cessation of medical treatment, refusal of life-support, relief of suffering and pain control that may hasten death, advance directives, and the powers of physicians to cease or authorize the cessation of medical treatment of incompetent, terminally ill patients.

Most significantly for our purposes, however, Section 5 of the Draft Bill submits three options for public debate and discussion regarding "active voluntary euthanasia." Option 1 is "the confirmation of the present legal position," which prohibits physician-assisted suicide and voluntary active euthanasia because arguments in favor of these practices do not provide sufficient grounds to weaken society's prohibition of intentional killing. Even though individual cases may present a strong case for assistance with dying, they cannot establish the foundation for a pro-euthanasia policy, a cornerstone of civilized society. Moreover, it would be impossible to establish sufficient safeguards to prevent abuse.

Option 2, "decision making by the medical practitioner," proposes legislation enabling a physician, upon satisfying certain conditions and meeting safeguards aimed at preventing abuse, to assist a patient with physician-assisted suicide or voluntary active euthanasia.

Option 3, "decision making by a panel or committee," proposes that "euthanasia" be regulated through legislation permitting a multi-disciplinary ethics committee to consider requests for euthanasia on the basis of set criteria.

The SALC should be commended for proposing options that give public debate a clear focus and contribute to the democratic process. Options 2 and 3 now accept the broader category of "intractable and unbearable illness" as an alternative to terminal illness, and the role of interpreters is now recognized, although physicians still remain the only persons empowered to assist with dying. Option 2 is confined to patients over the age of 18 years, but, significantly, the ethics-committee approach does not have this limitation.

Both Options 2 and 3 seem to propose legalizing physician-assisted suicide as well as voluntary active euthanasia. Option 2 refers to a physician making an end to a patient's suffering (voluntary active euthanasia), and enabling a patient to make an end to his or her suffering (physician-assisted suicide). In contrast, Option 3 refers to "euthanasia," which, presumably, includes both physician-assisted suicide and voluntary active euthanasia, although, the term "euthanasia" is still not defined in the Draft Bill. Whereas I have argued that there is no intrinsic moral difference between the practices of physician-assisted suicide and voluntary active euthanasia, both being forms of assistance with dying, in the political arena it may still be preferable to reach a compromise by legalizing physician-assisted suicide only, rather than insisting on legalizing both physician-assisted suicide and voluntary active euthanasia and getting no legislation passed.

The debate about Option 1, that legally prohibits physician-assisted suicide and voluntary active euthanasia, will have to be sensitive to credible empirical evidence. First, what reason do we have for claiming that legalizing assistance with dying would weaken society's prohibition of intentional killing, and thus undermine the law and good social relationships? Given its humane and strictly limited context, assistance with dying would seem *prima facie* less likely to do so, if at all, than executions, or killing in self-defense or war, none of which appears to have had these profound consequences. Second, what firm grounds, rather than speculation, do we have for the necessary inefficacy of safeguards?

Option 2 poses two further points for clarification or debate. First, its wording, namely that a physician "shall give effect to the request," may suggest that physicians have no choice but to honor the patient's request for physician-assisted suicide/voluntary active euthanasia if the conditions are met. By contrast, Option 3 and South Africa's abortion legislation[8] state that a physician "may" act on a patient's request, thus affirming an implicit conscience clause. Second, Option 2 does not mention mental or dementing illness. Again, this is a difficult question of consistency and justice, and as such worthy of public debate.

Option 3 may, in the political process, turn out to be a good compromise proposal. However, it introduces new difficulties. First, who would constitute an ethics committee and how would it function? Who elects or appoints the committee? Could someone who is in principle opposed to physician-assisted suicide/voluntary active euthanasia serve on such a committee? How would decisions be taken, for example, by majority vote or consensus? Second, should there not be provision made for appeal against the decision of an ethics committee? Third, and most significantly, it raises issues of distributive justice.[11] Since a committee approach is premised on the availability of additional resources, it could lead to discrimination against patients in areas with poor access to health-care facilities. Ethics committees, whose membership requires, among others, two physicians, a lawyer, and a member of a multi-disciplinary team, are likely to be limited to tertiary, and therefore urban, centres while rural areas may not have an "ethics capacity."

In the final analysis, Option 2 is preferable over Option 3, since an ethics committee would be an unjustifiably paternalistic institution that would take control away from the patient and physician and give it to a group of "outsiders." Attending physicians can exert the same caution and circumspection as a committee and, together with patients, they would be able to focus on the tragic choices at hand, while avoiding general debates about the morality of an already legalized practice, which may be the fate of an ethics-committee approach.

I thank Lesley Henley (University of Cape Town) and John Moskop (East Carolina University) for helpful comments during the preparation of this manuscript.

East Carolina University
Greenville, North Carolina

NOTES

[1] South African Law Commission Act, 19 of 1973.
[2] References in the text are to the numbered paragraphs of the Discussion Paper (SALC, 1997).
[3] Constitution of the Republic of South Africa Act, 108 of 1996.
[4] Since the first democratic election of 1994, many areas of public life have been transformed radically, for example, the liberalization of labor law, the introduction of the first stage of a national health service committed to universal access, the legalization of abortion, and the abolition of capital punishment. And, of course, it is in itself significant that the Commission found good reason to open a public debate on physician-assisted suicide and voluntary active euthanasia.
[5] The Commission rejects involuntary euthanasia (3.92), and suggests two alternative approaches to non-voluntary euthanasia, namely, enabling the courts to order only the cessation of medical treatment (4.120), or both the cessation of medical treatment and the termination of life (4.125).
[6] An interesting question is whether the option of terminal sedation makes physician-assisted suicide (and presumably also voluntary active euthanasia) redundant, as implied by some US Supreme Court judges in *Washington v. Glucksburg* 117 S. Ct. 2302 (1997). Whatever the case, some patients may justifiably prefer not to be terminally sedated.
[7] This constitutional (as opposed to moral) point was suggested to me in personal communication by Barney Sneiderman (Faculty of Law, University of Manitoba).
[8] Choice on Termination of Pregnancy Act, 92 of 1996.
[9] Child Care Act, 74 of 1983.
[10] *Soobramoney v. Minister of Health (Kwazulu-Natal)* CCT 32/97 (27 November 1997).
[11] This point was suggested to me in personal communication by Lesley D. Henley (Department of Paediatrics, Institute of Child Health, Red Cross War Memorial Children's Hospital, Cape Town).
[12] In Oregon's Death With Dignity Act, Or. Rev. Stat, Secs. 127.00 et seq. (1995) this period is 15 days (S 3.06). I do not know what exactly would constitute a reasonable period, but 15 days does seem to be a long time for someone whose suffering is extreme.
[13] 88% of S.A. physicians practice in urban areas (SAHR, 1998: ch. 5).

REFERENCES

Battin, M.P.: 1990, 'Seven caveats concerning the discussion of euthanasia in Holland', *Perspectives in Biology and Medicine* 34, pp. 73–80.

Battin, M.P.: 1991, 'Euthanasia: The way we do it, the way they do it', in T.A. Mappes and D. DeGrazia, (eds.), *Biomedical Ethics* (4th ed.), McGraw-Hill, New York, 1996, pp. 393–400.

Battin, M.P.: 1992, 'Voluntary euthanasia and the risks of abuse: can we learn anything from the Netherlands', *Law, Medicine and Health Care* 20, pp. 133–143.

Battin, M.P.: 1993, 'Seven (more) caveats concerning the discussion of euthanasia in the Netherlands', *APA Newsletters* 92, pp. 76–80.

Benatar, D., Benatar, S.R., Abratt, R. et al.: 1997, *Comments on the Draft Bill on End-of-Life Decisions,* Department of Medicine, University of Cape Town, Cape Town.

Brock, D.W.: 1987, 'Informed consent', in D. VanDeVeer and T. Regan (eds.), *Health Care Ethics,* Temple University Press, Philadelphia, pp. 98–126.

Brock, D.W.: 1992, 'Voluntary active euthanasia', *Hastings Center Report* 22, pp. 10–22.

Caplan, A.: 1998, 'Australia goes first', in A. Caplan, *Due Consideration: Controversy in the Age of Medical Miracles,* John Wiley, New York, pp. 225–226.

Chin, A.E., Hedberg, K., Higginson, G.K. et al.: 1999, 'Legalized physician-assisted suicide in Oregon – the first year's experience', *The New England Journal of Medicine* 340, pp. 577–583.

Dixon, N.: 1998, 'On the difference between physician-assisted suicide and active euthanasia', *Hastings Center Report* 28, pp. 25–29.

Doyal, L. and Henning, P.: 1994, 'Stopping treatment for end-stage renal failure: the rights of children and adolescents,' *Pediatric Nephrology* 8, pp. 768–771.

Dworkin, R.: 1997, 'Assisted suicide: what the court said', *New York Review of Books* XLIV(14) (September 25), pp. 40–44.

Foley, K. and Hendin, H.: 1999, 'The Oregon report: don't ask don't tell', *The Hastings Center Report* (May–June), pp. 37–42.

Foot, P.: 1977, 'Euthanasia', *Philosophy and Public Affairs* 6, pp. 85–112.

Freyer, D.R.: 1992, 'Children with cancer: special considerations in the discontinuation of life-sustaining treatment', *Medical and Pediatric Oncology* 20, pp. 136–142.

Kuhse, H.: 1991, 'Euthanasia', in P. Singer (ed.), *A Companion to Ethics,* Basil Blackwell, Oxford, pp. 294–302.

Landman W.A.: 1997, 'The ethics of physician-assisted suicide and euthanasia', *South African Medical Journal* 87, pp. 866–869.

Landman W.A.: 1998, 'Physician-assisted suicide and voluntary euthanasia - a response', *South African Medical Journal* 88, pp. 242–243.

Leichtentritt, R.D., Rettig, K.D., Miles, S.: 1999, 'Holocaust survivors' perspectives on the euthanasia debate', *Social Science and Medicine* 48, pp. 185–196.

MacFarlane, J.M.: 1997, 'Death and dying in Australia – some medico-legal problems for legislators', *Medicine and Law* 16, pp. 179–186.

Mackie, J.L.: 1974, *The Cement of the Universe: A Study of Causation,* Clarendon Press, Oxford.

Quill, T.E., Cassel, C.K., Meier, D.E.: 1992, 'Care of the hopelessly ill: proposed clinical criteria for physician-assisted suicide', *New England Journal of Medicine,* 327, pp. 1381–1383.

South African Health Review, 1998 (SAHR). http://www.hst.org.za/sahr

South African Law Commission (SALC): 1997, Discussion Paper 71, Project 86, *Euthanasia and the Artificial Preservation of Life,* Pretoria, South Africa. http://www.law.wits.ac.za/salc/discussn/dp71.html

South African Law Commission (SALC): 1998, Issue Paper 13, Project 110, The Review of the Child Care Act, First Issue Paper, Pretoria, South Africa. http://www.law.wits.ac.za/salc/issue/ip13.html

South African Law Commission (SALC): 1999, Project 86, Euthanasia and the Artificial Preservation of Life, Pretoria, South Africa. http://www.law.wits.ac.za/salc/report/euthansum.html

Turner, J.S., Michell, W.L., Morgan, C.J. et al.: 1996, 'Limitation of life support: frequency and practice in a London and a Cape Town intensive care unit', *Intensive Care Medicine* 22, pp. 1020–1025.

van der Maas, P.J., van der Wal, G., Haverkate, I. et al.: 1996, 'Euthanasia, physician-assisted suicide, and other medical practices involving the end of life in the Netherlands, 1990–1995', *New England Journal of Medicine* 335, pp. 1699–1705.

van der Wal, G., van der Maas, P.J., Bosma, J.M. et al.: 1996, 'Evaluation of the notification procedure for physician-assisted death in the Netherlands,' *New England Journal of Medicine* 335, pp. 1706–1711.

Wharton, R.H., Levine, K.R., Buka, S. et al.: 1996, 'Advance care planning for children with special needs: a survey of parental attitudes', *Pediatrics* 97, pp. 682–687.

NOTES ON CONTRIBUTORS

Margaret P. Battin is Professor of Philosophy and Adjunct Professor of Internal Medicine, Division of Medical Ethics, at the University of Utah. She is a graduate of Bryn Mawr College, and holds a M.F.A. in fiction writing and a Ph.D. in philosophy from the University of California at Irvine. The author of prize-winning short stories, she has also authored, edited, or co-edited twelve books, among them a study of philosophical issues in suicide; a scholarly edition of John Donne's *Biathanatos;* a collection on age-rationing of medical care; *Puzzles About Art*, a volume of case-puzzles in aesthetics; a text on professional ethics; and *Ethics in the Sanctuary,* a study of ethical issues in organized religion. A collection of her essays on end-of-life issues written over the last fifteen years is entitled *The Least Worst Death.* She has been engaged in research on active euthanasia and assisted suicide in the Netherlands. She has also recently published *Ethical Issues in Suicide,* trade-titled *The Death Debate*, as well as several co-edited collections, including *Drug Use in Euthanasia and Assisted Suicide* and *Physician-Assisted Suicide: Expanding the Debate.* Just published in 1999 is *Praying for a Cure,* a jointly authored volume on the ethics of religious refusal of medical treatment. She is currently at work on a book on world population growth and reproductive rights, and on a sourcebook on ethical issues in suicide.

Dan W. Brock is Charles C. Tillinghast, Jr. University Professor, Professor of Philosophy and Biomedical Ethics, and Director of the Center for Biomedical Ethics at Brown University where he has taught since 1969. He received his B.A. in economics from Cornell University and his Ph.D. in philosophy from Columbia University. He served as Staff Philosopher on the President's Commission for the Study of Ethical Problems in Medicine in 1981-1982, was a member of the Ethics Working Group of the Clinton Task Force on National Health Reform in 1993, and was President of the American Association of Bioethics in 1995-96. He is author of over 130 published papers in bioethics and moral and political philosophy, and of *Deciding for Others: The Ethics of Surrogate Decision Making* (1989, with Allen E. Buchanan), *Life and Death: Philosophical Essays in Biomedical Ethics* (1993), and *From Chance to Choice:*

Loretta M. Kopelman and Kenneth A. De Ville (eds.), Physician-Assisted Suicide, 227–230.
© 2001 *Kluwer Academic Publishers. Printed in Great Britain.*

Genetics and Justice (with Allen Buchanan, Norman Daniels and Daniel Wikler.

Kenneth De Ville is Professor, Department of Medical Humanities, Brody School of Medicine at East Carolina University. He received his doctorate from Rice University in 1989 and his law degree from the University of Texas in 1992. De Ville is author of the book *Medical Malpractice in Nineteenth Century America: Origins and Legacy* (1990). His articles have appeared in such journals as: the *American Journal of Public Health*, the *Journal of Law, Medicine and Ethics*, *Theoretical Medicine & Bioethics*, *The Historian*, the *Journal of Clinical Ethics*, *Seminars in Pediatric Surgery*, *Pediatrics*, *Trends in Health Care, Law & Ethics*, *HEC Forum*, *Current Surgery*, *Clinics in Obstetrics and Gynecology*, the *Missouri Law Review*, *Mount Sinai Medical Journal*, the *International Journal of Technology Assessment in Health Care*, the *Journal of Medicine and Philosophy*, the *Journal of Legal Medicine*, and *Defense Counsel Journal*. He is "Of Counsel" at Hollowell, Peacock & Meyer, P.A., Raleigh, N.C.

H. Tristram Engelhardt, Jr. is Professor in the Department of Medicine, Baylor College of Medicine, and Professor in the Department of Philosophy, Rice University, and a member of the Center for Medical Ethics and Health Policy. He is Editor of *The Journal of Medicine and Philosophy* and of the book series, *Philosophical Studies in Contemporary Culture*. He is also co-editor of the journal *Christian Bioethics* and the book series *Clinical Medical Ethics*. *The Foundations of Bioethics* (1996) had just appeared in a thoroughly revised second edition.

Raymond G. Frey is Professor of Philosophy at Bowling Green State University and Senior Research Fellow in the Social Philosophy and Policy Center there. His graduate education was at the University of Virginia and Oxford University, from which he received his D. Phil. Degree. He has written numerous articles and books in moral and political philosophy and in 18th-century British moral philosophy. His most recent book is *Euthanasia and Physician-Assisted Suicide* (Cambridge University Press), jointly authored with Gerald Dworkin and Sissela Bok. Forthcoming are books on suicide and on the moral philosophy of Butler, Shaftesbury, and Hume.

Robert L. Holmes is Professor of Philosophy at the University of Rochester. He is author of *Basic Moral Philosophy, On War and Morality, Frankena on Is and Ought, Perspectives on Morality and War in American Society: A Symposium,* and editor of *Nonviolence in Theory and Practice.* His research interests are ethics, social philosophy & philosophy of war.

Willem A. Landman is CEO, Ethics Institute of South Africa, Pretoria, SA. He was formerly Professor of Medical Humanities in The Brody School of Medicine at East Carolina University in Greenville, North Carolina. He was a South Africa-at-Large Rhodes Scholar at the Oxford University, where he read philosophy and theology. He received his D. Phil. (political philosophy) degree from the University of Stellenbosch, and holds a law degree from the University of South Africa. He was chair of philosophy departments at the Universities of Transkei and the Western Cape. He has published journal articles on issues in the philosophy of religion, moral philosophy, and bioethics.

Loretta M. Kopelman is professor and founding chair of the Department of Medical Humanities at The Brody School of Medicine at East Carolina University. She has published over 100 book chapters and articles and is a member of the Editorial Board of The *Journal of Medicine and Philosophy, Medical Humanities:* edition of the *Journal of Medical Ethics.* She was President of the Society for Health and Human Values, and founding President of the American Society of Bioethics and Humanities. She served on the Editorial Board of the *Encyclopedia of Bioethics,* second edition. Her publications reflect her interest in the rights and welfare of patients and research subjects, including children and vulnerable populations, death and dying, moral problems in psychiatry, research ethics and other issues in philosophy of medicine and bioethics. She has edited *The Rights of Children and Retarded Persons, Ethics and Mental Retardation, Children and Health Care: Moral and Social Issues,* and *Building Bioethics: Conversations with Clouser and Friends.*

Steven Miles is a geriatrician and medical ethicist. He practices and teaches geriatric internal medicine in nursing homes, clinics and hospitals. He is Associate Professor of Internal Medicine in the Department of Medicine and Division of Geriatric Medicine at the University of Minnesota and St. Paul Ramsey Medical Center. He is faculty at the

Center for Bioethics, the Center for Advances Feminist Studies, and the University Council on Aging at the University of Minnesota. He has published more than 100 peer reviewed articles and lectured extensively on end-of-life care, nursing home care, medical education, medical ethics, and health care reform. He is President of the American Association of Bioethics.

David Resnik is an Associate Professor of Medical Humanities at The Brody School of Medicine at East Carolina University. He has a Ph.D. (1990) and MA (1987) in Philosophy from the University of North Carolina at Chapel Hill, and a BA (1985) in Philosophy from Davidson College. He has published over 40 articles on various topics in the philosophy of science and ethics and is the author of *The Ethics of Science: an Introduction* (Routledge, 1998), and a co-author (with Pamela Langer and Holly Steinkraus) of *Human Germ-line Gene Therapy: Scientific, Moral, and Political Issues* (RG Landes, 1999). His research interests include ethical issues in science, ethical issues in human genetics, biomedical ethics, and the philosophy of biology and medicine.

Gail Povar is a practicing internist in Silver Spring, Maryland and Clinical Professor of Medicine at the George Washington University School of Medicine and Health Sciences. Dr. Povar has written widely in the fields of preventive medicine and medical ethics. She is co-author of the book *Striving for Quality in Health Care*, co-edited *Putting Prevention into Practice*, co-authored with Janet Bickel the article "Women in Medicine" in the current edition of the *Encyclopedia of Bioethics*, and has published numerous articles and book chapters. She is on the editorial board of the *Journal of Clinical Ethics*. Dr. Povar has served as a consultant to both the Institute of Medicine and the National Institutes of Health, and has been chair of the George Washington University Hospital Ethics Committee since 1987.

Laurie Zoloth is Associate Professor of Social Ethics and Jewish Philosophy, and Director of the Program in Jewish Studies at San Francisco State University. Her books include *Health Care and the Ethics of Encounter: A Jewish Discussion of Justice*, *Notes From a Narrow Ridge: Bioethics and Religion*, co-edited with Dena Davis, and *The Margin of Error: The Inevitability, Necessity and Ethics of Mistakes in Medicine and Bioethics*, co-edited with Susan Rubin.

INDEX

Philosophy and Medicine

1. H. Tristram Engelhardt, Jr. and S.F. Spicker (eds.): *Evaluation and Explanation in the Biomedical Sciences.* 1975   ISBN 90-277-0553-4
2. S.F. Spicker and H. Tristram Engelhardt, Jr. (eds.): *Philosophical Dimensions of the Neuro-Medical Sciences.* 1976   ISBN 90-277-0672-7
3. S.F. Spicker and H. Tristram Engelhardt, Jr. (eds.): *Philosophical Medical Ethics.* Its Nature and Significance. 1977   ISBN 90-277-0772-3
4. H. Tristram Engelhardt, Jr. and S.F. Spicker (eds.): *Mental Health.* Philosophical Perspectives. 1978   ISBN 90-277-0828-2
5. B.A. Brody and H. Tristram Engelhardt, Jr. (eds.): *Mental Illness.* Law and Public Policy. 1980   ISBN 90-277-1057-0
6. H. Tristram Engelhardt, Jr., S.F. Spicker and B. Towers (eds.): *Clinical Judgment.* A Critical Appraisal. 1979   ISBN 90-277-0952-1
7. S.F. Spicker (ed.): *Organism, Medicine, and Metaphysics.* Essays in Honor of Hans Jonas on His 75th Birthday. 1978   ISBN 90-277-0823-1
8. E.E. Shelp (ed.): *Justice and Health Care.* 1981
                    ISBN 90-277-1207-7; Pb 90-277-1251-4
9. S.F. Spicker, J.M. Healey, Jr. and H. Tristram Engelhardt, Jr. (eds.): *The Law-Medicine Relation.* A Philosophical Exploration. 1981   ISBN 90-277-1217-4
10. W.B. Bondeson, H. Tristram Engelhardt, Jr., S.F. Spicker and J.M. White, Jr. (eds.): *New Knowledge in the Biomedical Sciences.* Some Moral Implications of Its Acquisition, Possession, and Use. 1982   ISBN 90-277-1319-7
11. E.E. Shelp (ed.): *Beneficence and Health Care.* 1982   ISBN 90-277-1377-4
12. G.J. Agich (ed.): *Responsibility in Health Care.* 1982   ISBN 90-277-1417-7
13. W.B. Bondeson, H. Tristram Engelhardt, Jr., S.F. Spicker and D.H. Winship: *Abortion and the Status of the Fetus.* 2nd printing, 1984   ISBN 90-277-1493-2
14. E.E. Shelp (ed.): *The Clinical Encounter.* The Moral Fabric of the Patient-Physician Relationship. 1983   ISBN 90-277-1593-9
15. L. Kopelman and J.C. Moskop (eds.): *Ethics and Mental Retardation.* 1984
                    ISBN 90-277-1630-7
16. L. Nordenfelt and B.I.B. Lindahl (eds.): *Health, Disease, and Causal Explanations in Medicine.* 1984   ISBN 90-277-1660-9
17. E.E. Shelp (ed.): *Virtue and Medicine.* Explorations in the Character of Medicine. 1985   ISBN 90-277-1808-3
18. P. Carrick: *Medical Ethics in Antiquity.* Philosophical Perspectives on Abortion and Euthanasia. 1985   ISBN 90-277-1825-3; Pb 90-277-1915-2
19. J.C. Moskop and L. Kopelman (eds.): *Ethics and Critical Care Medicine.* 1985
                    ISBN 90-277-1820-2
20. E.E. Shelp (ed.): *Theology and Bioethics.* Exploring the Foundations and Frontiers. 1985   ISBN 90-277-1857-1

21. G.J. Agich and C.E. Begley (eds.): *The Price of Health.* 1986
ISBN 90-277-2285-4

22. E.E. Shelp (ed.): *Sexuality and Medicine.* Vol. I: Conceptual Roots. 1987
ISBN 90-277-2290-0; Pb 90-277-2386-9

23. E.E. Shelp (ed.): *Sexuality and Medicine.* Vol. II: Ethical Viewpoints in Transition. 1987 ISBN 1-55608-013-1; Pb 1-55608-016-6

24. R.C. McMillan, H. Tristram Engelhardt, Jr., and S.F. Spicker (eds.): *Euthanasia and the Newborn.* Conflicts Regarding Saving Lives. 1987
ISBN 90-277-2299-4; Pb 1-55608-039-5

25. S.F. Spicker, S.R. Ingman and I.R. Lawson (eds.): *Ethical Dimensions of Geriatric Care.* Value Conflicts for the 21th Century. 1987 ISBN 1-55608-027-1

26. L. Nordenfelt: *On the Nature of Health.* An Action-Theoretic Approach. 2nd, rev. ed. 1995 SBN 0-7923-3369-1; Pb 0-7923-3470-1

27. S.F. Spicker, W.B. Bondeson and H. Tristram Engelhardt, Jr. (eds.): *The Contraceptive Ethos.* Reproductive Rights and Responsibilities. 1987
ISBN 1-55608-035-2

28. S.F. Spicker, I. Alon, A. de Vries and H. Tristram Engelhardt, Jr. (eds.): *The Use of Human Beings in Research.* With Special Reference to Clinical Trials. 1988
ISBN 1-55608-043-3

29. N.M.P. King, L.R. Churchill and A.W. Cross (eds.): *The Physician as Captain of the Ship.* A Critical Reappraisal. 1988 ISBN 1-55608-044-1

30. H.-M. Sass and R.U. Massey (eds.): *Health Care Systems.* Moral Conflicts in European and American Public Policy. 1988 ISBN 1-55608-045-X

31. R.M. Zaner (ed.): *Death: Beyond Whole-Brain Criteria.* 1988
ISBN 1-55608-053-0

32. B.A. Brody (ed.): *Moral Theory and Moral Judgments in Medical Ethics.* 1988
ISBN 1-55608-060-3

33. L.M. Kopelman and J.C. Moskop (eds.): *Children and Health Care.* Moral and Social Issues. 1989 ISBN 1-55608-078-6

34. E.D. Pellegrino, J.P. Langan and J. Collins Harvey (eds.): *Catholic Perspectives on Medical Morals.* Foundational Issues. 1989 ISBN 1-55608-083-2

35. B.A. Brody (ed.): *Suicide and Euthanasia.* Historical and Contemporary Themes. 1989 ISBN 0-7923-0106-4

36. H.A.M.J. ten Have, G.K. Kimsma and S.F. Spicker (eds.): *The Growth of Medical Knowledge.* 1990 ISBN 0-7923-0736-4

37. I. Löwy (ed.): *The Polish School of Philosophy of Medicine.* From Tytus Chałubiński (1820–1889) to Ludwik Fleck (1896–1961). 1990
ISBN 0-7923-0958-8

38. T.J. Bole III and W.B. Bondeson: *Rights to Health Care.* 1991
ISBN 0-7923-1137-X

39. M.A.G. Cutter and E.E. Shelp (eds.): *Competency*. A Study of Informal Competency Determinations in Primary Care. 1991   ISBN 0-7923-1304-6
40. J.L. Peset and D. Gracia (eds.): *The Ethics of Diagnosis*. 1992
          ISBN 0-7923-1544-8
41. K.W. Wildes, S.J., F. Abel, S.J. and J.C. Harvey (eds.): *Birth, Suffering, and Death*. Catholic Perspectives at the Edges of Life. 1992 [CSiB-1]
          ISBN 0-7923-1547-2; Pb 0-7923-2545-1
42. S.K. Toombs: *The Meaning of Illness*. A Phenomenological Account of the Different Perspectives of Physician and Patient. 1992
          ISBN 0-7923-1570-7; Pb 0-7923-2443-9
43. D. Leder (ed.): *The Body in Medical Thought and Practice*. 1992
          ISBN 0-7923-1657-6
44. C. Delkeskamp-Hayes and M.A.G. Cutter (eds.): *Science, Technology, and the Art of Medicine*. European-American Dialogues. 1993   ISBN 0-7923-1869-2
45. R. Baker, D. Porter and R. Porter (eds.): *The Codification of Medical Morality*. Historical and Philosophical Studies of the Formalization of Western Medical Morality in the 18th and 19th Centuries, Volume One: Medical Ethics and Etiquette in the 18th Century. 1993   ISBN 0-7923-1921-4
46. K. Bayertz (ed.): *The Concept of Moral Consensus*. The Case of Technological Interventions in Human Reproduction. 1994   ISBN 0-7923-2615-6
47. L. Nordenfelt (ed.): *Concepts and Measurement of Quality of Life in Health Care*. 1994 [ESiP-1]   ISBN 0-7923-2824-8
48. R. Baker and M.A. Strosberg (eds.) with the assistance of J. Bynum: *Legislating Medical Ethics*. A Study of the New York State Do-Not-Resuscitate Law. 1995
          ISBN 0-7923-2995-3
49. R. Baker (ed.): *The Codification of Medical Morality*. Historical and Philosophical Studies of the Formalization of Western Morality in the 18th and 19th Centuries, Volume Two: Anglo-American Medical Ethics and Medical Jurisprudence in the 19th Century. 1995   ISBN 0-7923-3528-7; Pb 0-7923-3529-5
50. R.A. Carson and C.R. Burns (eds.): *Philosophy of Medicine and Bioethics*. A Twenty-Year Retrospective and Critical Appraisal. 1997 ISBN 0-7923-3545-7
51. K.W. Wildes, S.J. (ed.): *Critical Choices and Critical Care*. Catholic Perspectives on Allocating Resources in Intensive Care Medicine. 1995 [CSiB-2]
          ISBN 0-7923-3382-9
52. K. Bayertz (ed.): *Sanctity of Life and Human Dignity*. 1996
          ISBN 0-7923-3739-5
53. Kevin Wm. Wildes, S.J. (ed.): *Infertility: A Crossroad of Faith, Medicine, and Technology*. 1996   ISBN 0-7923-4061-2
54. Kazumasa Hoshino (ed.): *Japanese and Western Bioethics*. Studies in Moral Diversity. 1996   ISBN 0-7923-4112-0

Philosophy and Medicine

55. E. Agius and S. Busuttil (eds.): *Germ-Line Intervention and our Responsibilities to Future Generations.* 1998   ISBN 0-7923-4828-1
56. L.B. McCullough: *John Gregory and the Invention of Professional Medical Ethics and the Professional Medical Ethics and the Profession of Medicine.* 1998
                    ISBN 0-7923-4917-2
57. L.B. McCullough: *John Gregory's Writing on Medical Ethics and Philosophy of Medicine.* 1998 [CiME-1]   ISBN 0-7923-5000-6
58. H.A.M.J. ten Have and H.-M. Sass (eds.): *Consensus Formation in Healthcare Ethics.* 1998 [ESiP-2]   ISBN 0-7923-4944-X
59. H.A.M.J. ten Have and J.V.M. Welie (eds.): *Ownership of the Human Body.* Philosophical Considerations on the Use of the Human Body and its Parts in Healthcare. 1998 [ESiP-3]   ISBN 0-7923-5150-9
60. M.J. Cherry (ed.): *Persons and Their Bodies.* Rights, Responsibilities, Relationships. 1999   ISBN 0-7923-5701-9
61. R. Fan (ed.): *Confucian Bioethics.* 1999 [APSiB-1]   ISBN 0-7923-5853-8
62. L.M. Kopelman (ed.): *Building Bioethics.* Conversations with Clouser and Friends on Medical Ethics. 1999   ISBN 0-7923-5853-8
63. W.E. Stempsey: *Disease and Diagnosis.* 2000   PB ISBN 0-7923-6322-1
64. H.T. Engelhardt (ed.): *The Philosophy of Medicine.* Framing the Field. 2000
                    ISBN 0-7923-6223-3
65. S. Wear, J.J. Bono, G. Logue and A. McEvoy (eds.): *Ethical Issues in Health Care on the Frontiers of the Twenty-First Century.* 2000   ISBN 0-7923-6277-2
66. M. Potts, P.A. Byrne and R.G. Nilges (eds.): *Beyond Brain Death.* The Case Against Brain Based Criteria for Human Death. 2000   ISBN 0-7923-6578-X
67. L.M. Kopelman and K.A. De Ville (eds.): *Physician-Assisted Suicide.* What are the Issues? 2001   ISBN -7923-7142-9

KLUWER ACADEMIC PUBLISHERS – DORDRECHT / BOSTON / LONDON